The Metabolism
Plan
WORKBOOK

2021 Edition

ALSO BY LYN-GENET RECITAS

The Plan

The Plan Cookbook

The Metabolism Plan

The Metabolism Plan Vegan and Vegetarian Cookbook

The Metabolism
Plan
WORKBOOK

2021 Edition

LYN-GENET RECITAS,

HHP- Executive Director of Nutrition

New York Times
bestselling author of
The Plan and *The Metabolism Plan*

Lyn-Genet Press

New York

The advice herein is not intended to replace the services of trained health professionals or to be a substitute for medical advice. You are advised to consult with your healthcare professional with regard to matters relating to your health and, in particular, regarding matters that may require diagnosis or medical attention.

Lyn-Genet Press

Post Office Box 474

Dobbs Ferry, NY 10522

lyngenet.com

Printed in the United States of America

First Edition: September 2021

10 9 8 7 6 5 4 3 2 1

Names: Recitas, Lyn-Genet, author.
Title: The Metabolism Plan Workbook: 2021 Edition / Lyn-Genet Recitas, *New York Times* bestselling author of *The Plan* and *The Metabolism Plan*.
Description: First Edition. | Lyn-Genet Press, 2021.
Identifiers: LCCN: 2018911271 | ISBN 978-1-7328165-2-7 (paperback) | ISBN 978-1-7328165-3-4 (ebook)
Subjects: BISAC: HEALTH & FITNESS / Diet & Nutrition / Weight Loss

Table of Contents

Introduction

It's not working anymore

You are so frustrated, right?

All the diets, all the tricks, all the time in the gym, everything that used to work doesn't work anymore. You're doing everything "right". So, what's wrong?

Your best friend loses weight in a spinning class, and you gain a pound. Your brother can eat pizza and hotdogs and be skinny as a rail, and you're dutifully eating salads and cauliflower. MISERABLE because you just won't stop gaining weight.

I get it, I really do, and I'm here to help. This workbook is for you. Well actually it's for everybody because this is not a diet! It's about you being your healthiest. When you eat the foods that work for YOUR body, and yes, that may include grilled cheese and fries, you will be at your best weight and your best health.

The two go hand in hand. Remember you will always be at your best weight when you are HEALTHY.

I'm here to help you understand what foods and exercise your beautiful unique body wants. So, I want you to stop listening to the "experts", and instead listen to the person that knows your body better than any trainer or nutritionist. You. I am going to teach you to listen to YOUR body.

I remember one client telling me she hated oranges growing up and would ask her mom for a cookie for a treat. Guess what? She was highly reactive to oranges and listening to her body. So, we need to relearn how to communicate and listen to what our body is telling us. Guess what? The scale, the thing you dread stepping on, is a super reliable way to track what your body loves. And what it doesn't.

Let's say you spend the day eating salmon, cauliflower rice and green juices. The next day you are FRUSTRATED because you have GAINED weight!! How could that happen?

Gaining weight to healthy foods is very common. That number on the scale? That's just your chemical response to food. When you gain weight with healthy food that's a histamine response that your body elicits when it is exposed to a reactive food. A reactive food is a food that causes inflammation and weight gain. You may have heard that there are foods that produce histamine. But the fact is there is no universal histamine producing foods. There are only the foods that are reactive for you which elicit a histamine response.

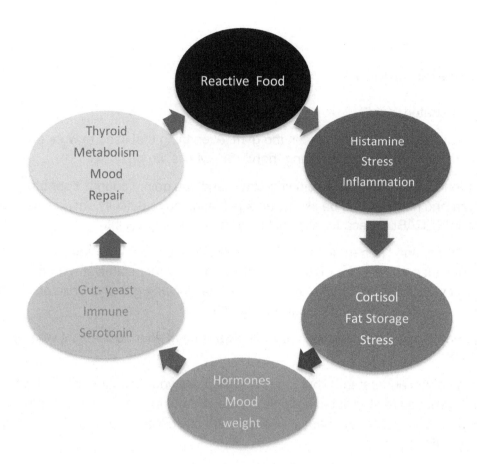

G.A- 49- "Thank you Lyn-Genet Recitas for educating me how I can have fun eating healthy and still lose unwanted pounds without the drama of cringing before getting on the scale. To accomplish this goal, however, requires a plan...., The Plan.

This book not only changed my perspective about eating foods packed with nutrients, but it has been years since I felt so alive and guilt free eating basic meals. I feel fantastic inside out, and I lose the weight without taking a single vitamin or going to the gym. Lyn-Genet was right when she said the scale will become your best friend, because it has. For the first time EVER, I am no longer scared to eat the foods I love, because I know how to test whether or not my body is reactive/non-reactive to certain foods and what I need to do to balance the playing field.

I highly recommend this book to anyone who is seriously committed to wanting to feel good in their body. No more trying one diet after another, only to lose the weight and gain it all back (and some more) for me.

A heartfelt thank you to Lyn-Genet Recitas for your guidance to good eating and awesome health."

So, let's start to uncover some of the "healthy" things you are doing which is keeping you from your health and weight goals!

Histamine

What is histamine? You can read more about it in my books The Plan and The Metabolism Plan. But this workbook is a quick synopsis of my two nutrition books.

Basically, histamine is your capillaries leaking fluid. It could be seasonal allergies. Or it could be the foods you are eating. Histamine triggers this negative feedback loops you see above.

This illustrates how much an inflammatory food can affect every part of our overall health and mood.

Find the foods that work for you and so many health and weight issues will be resolved.

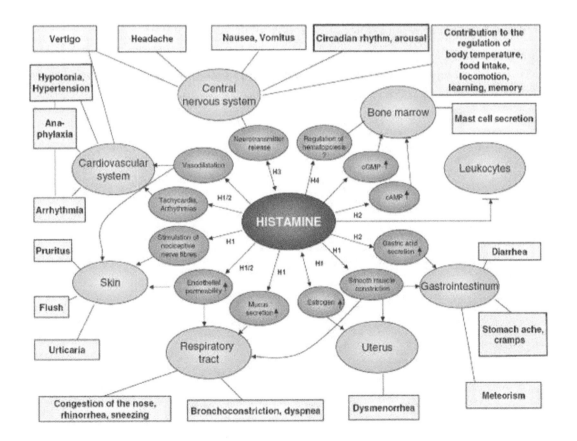

Finding Your Balance

I am a chef and I love food! I also run two businesses and I'm a mom. I get it, relearning everything you've been thru can seem overwhelming, but I promise you, if you put in 30 days you *are going* to find the roadmap for a happy healthy life, full of joyous food.

You see it's not the fun of foods that I'm worried about. These foods are a treat, and you deserve to have fun foods occasionally.

It's those darn healthy foods you are dutifully eating (and not always enjoying) that concern me. Turkey, asparagus, quinoa, Greek yogurt, red peppers, black beans. High reactive? Yes, in fact 85% of the population over 35 may react to these foods.

Shocking right? And the list of foods you are SUPPOSED to eat to lose weight and lower inflammation that are not working for you goes on. These "healthy" foods will also eventually affect your health. Your body is being kind to you when you gain weight from a food that is inflammatory. But if you don't listen to the symptoms of weight gain it eventually becomes a health issue.

So, I want you to think of this process – weight gain from "clean" foods- as your body saying, "I love you". If the cauliflower causes weight gain and the potato doesn't, eat the potato. If shrimp causes weight gain, but the halibut doesn't, eat that.

Here are some of the surprising foods that are keeping you from your health and weight goals. This is why I say everyone is eating at least a few healthy foods that are causing inflammation. What foods on this list do you eat?

85%+ Reactive
- Shrimp
- Turkey
- Canned tomato sauce
- Eggplant
- Oatmeal
- Greek yogurt
- Black beans
- Cannellini beans
- Cauliflower
- Cabbage
- Hard-boiled eggs
- Roasted nuts
- Salmon
- Asparagus
- Bagels
- Farm raised fish
- Deli Meats-regular sodium
- Sushi with sauces
- Veal
- Strawberries
- Artichokes
- Pistachios

70% Reactive
- Yogurt, regular
- Green beans
- Pasta
- Bananas
- Roasted Nut Butter
- Walnuts
- Green peppers
- Pineapple
- Tofu
- Bok choy- broccolini
- Tuna
- Green juices
- Protein powders

60% Reactive
- Red Peppers
- Mushrooms (excluding shiitake)
- Pork

60% Reactive (cont.)
- Grapefruit
- Quinoa
- Oranges
- Melon (except watermelon)
- Tahini
- Mahi, snapper
- Almond milk

50% Reactive
- Cow's milk
- Couscous
- White rice
- Tomatoes
- Edamame
- Brussels

40% Reactive
- Pintos
- Whole Eggs
- Cashews

30% Reactive
- Parmesan
- Flounder/Halibut
- Scallops
- Lentils

20% Reactive
- Sourdough Bread
- Snow Peas
- Winter Squash
- Crab
- Tempeh
- Butternut Squash
- Duck
- Potatoes
- Snow peas
- Pecans

10% or less reactive
- Avocado
- Mango
- Garlic
- Onions
- Shiitaki mushrooms *(may be higher if you have yeast)*
- Radicchio
- Endive
- Lamb
- Chicken
- Goat or sheep's cheese
- Pears
- Broccoli
- Carrots
- Kale
- Zucchini
- Beets
- Steak
- Sunflower Seeds
- Pumpkin Seeds
- Raw Almonds
- Apples
- Pears
- Blueberries
- Chia Seeds
- Frisee
- Coconut Milk
- Rice Milk
- Basmati Rice
- Fennel
- Coconut flour
- Beef
- Endive
- Escarole
- Yellow Squash
- Organic spinach

TU 53, "Much more a food protocol than a diet: I love this book. It is simple and doesn't spend a lot of time arguing with you about "THIS "being bad and "THAT" being bad. In fact, Recitas seems to love food and wants you to enjoy it as much as possible. I also like that it starts off immediately addressing foods in the "healthy "eating category that are most of us who eat well are already familiar with. That some of these foods can be the "culprit" is the place where I hear the most heated discussions! It is shocking to now consider that though we can eat healthy and exercise, the very healthy foods we are eating to solve the issues, may be backfiring in our own systems. I have personally had many people buy the book after hearing about the Plan from me because, like me, we all are having significant health issues, mostly of an inflammatory nature. (Most of us are over 50) Some of us now talking about THE PLAN are now looking at the INFLAMMATION aspects of our conditions for the first time. That is true for me. I like to see that LOSING WEIGHT is JUST A SIDE BENEFIT. I love the way Recitas has us looking at weight as "DATA" and seeing our weight as a mere tool to help us in maintaining personal health. FOR THOSE OF YOU WITH THYROID issues, this PLAN is really interesting. In fact, for those of us who never before thought we HAD a thyroid issue, this can be a wakeup call. When the ladies I know started talking about the PLAN there were numbers of them who started to wonder if thyroid was an issue and generally this has ended up with them finding out that it is true, and they want to use The Plan rather than meds (IF they can) to address the problems.

The real issue that comes up again and again is "This must be just another ELIMINATION health plan". I think Lyn could stand to talk more about those differences since people who have invested hundreds and even thousands of dollars into all of this may find The Plan just TOO simple! They just see The Plan it as exactly what they are doing and but studying the book and reading I can now see it sure isn't always so!

All in all THE PLAN is stirring discussion on a wide variety of issues related to general health and understanding that losing weight is really only a BONUS you get from letting your body heal and now help you be well. BRAVO Lyn!

Exercise

Those hour-long classes or workout videos that you're struggling to get into, stressing yourself out about, may be the reason why you are gaining 5 to 10 pounds every year. You see we have been taught that the harder we go the better off we will be but, in fact they can be the exact opposite.

Most people don't need more than 8 to 20 minutes of exercise every other day to be lean and fit and strong. Are some folks genetically programmed to be athletes? Absolutely. Do you fall into this category? Probably not.

So, it's time for you to stop trying to take a square peg and fit it in a round hole. Instead, what I want you to do is find what works for your body. I can tell you right now- trying to follow all of these rules that are built for somebody else is increasing your stress and your waistline.

So, let's delve deeper into why diets and most exercise programs don't work especially over the age of 40.

SH- age 50- I should point out that I'm a reformed Spinning addict, a very educated eater, and I love to cook with real ingredients. That being said, I love this book. I was a client of Lyn's back in 2010 and just restarted my Planning lifestyle this year after the birth of my 2nd daughter. This book and her appearance on Dr. Oz were perfectly timed. The book gives you all the information you need to make comprehensive decisions and understand your outcomes. I was a one-on-one client of Lyn's back in 2010, and I can tell you this book answers all the questions I used to harass her with via email and texts (I was a very "interactive" client - LOL!). As a result of being on The Plan the first time around, I lost 23 lbs effortlessly, and this was at 39 y/o with baby weight from my then 4-year-old (yeah, I know - it wasn't baby weight anymore). After the birth of my 2nd child, the holidays, and everyday time crunches, my eating habits were less than stellar, and I could tell from my skin, energy output, and sleeplessness that I needed to recalibrate. Since restarting The Plan last week, I felt 100% better by Day 3. I no longer have lower back pain when I sat up in bed

> *for prolonged periods, I could actually bend to tie my shoes without that "tight" feeling in my knees, and I spring out of bed in the mornings. On the days you discover no reactivity to the previous day's menu, you're happy dancing in the street, and the days you realize you're reactive to a menu item, you're stashing that info in your arsenal so you don't make that mistake again. Either way you win, and in the end, you're steering your own success.*

How The Plan Works

The Plan is the most reliable way of finding the healthy foods that can cause inflammation, make you overweight and hasten the aging process. Wait- healthy foods make you fat? I know it's counterintuitive, but it's true. Healthy, low-calorie foods like green beans, strawberries, or oatmeal can cause one to two-pound weight gain. Up to 85% of the people that have worked with us at The Plan experience exponential weight gain to these healthy foods – up to four pounds!

This doesn't make sense, it's a calorie in, a calorie out, right?

Wrong.

Well, then how does this happen? The simplest answer is that these foods can trigger an inflammatory response. This inflammatory response triggers a domino effect that ultimately affects your immune system. That "healthy" spinach and egg white omelette may be prematurely aging you, expanding your waistline and cause your health to decline.

I've written 4 books published in 15 languages that have helped people all over the world reduce inflammation and lose weight quickly. This workbook in conjunction with The Metabolism Plan is going to help you find the foods and exercises that work best for your body

What you need to know is that you are chemically unique; your weight and your health are just Your chemical reactions to food.

You also need to remember that aging is a state of inflammation and systems start to slow down as we get older. Your body just can't repair as quickly as it did in your teens and twenties. Digestive enzyme production slows down, stomach acid and saliva decreases, all of which aid digestion. Hormonal imbalances trigger yeast flareups which changes our gut flora and our hormones. The foods you used to be able to break down easily when we were younger are just harder to break down in our thirties, forties and fifties and beyond.

When you eat a healthy food that doesn't work for YOUR chemistry there are many systems that are impacted, and this inflammatory response can last for 72 hours.

Histamine is released, and cortisol levels rise controlling long term fat storage. Increased cortisol production negatively impacts hormones such as progesterone and testosterone.

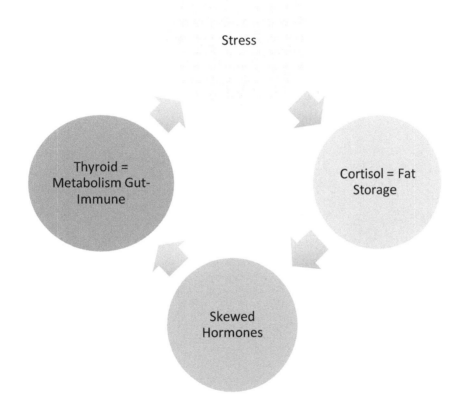

The Metabolism Myth

Does your metabolism really slow as you age?

Thank goodness the answer is no! But what is true is that certain factors can facilitate a metabolic slow down and that's why I'm here. I am going to help you understand the factors that are affecting you and your thyroid.

Many people don't realize this, but the thyroid is the master gland for your metabolism and anything that has a negative effect on it will slow the rate at which you lose weight and heal.

So you now know this is the breakdown of what happens when you eat a reactive food

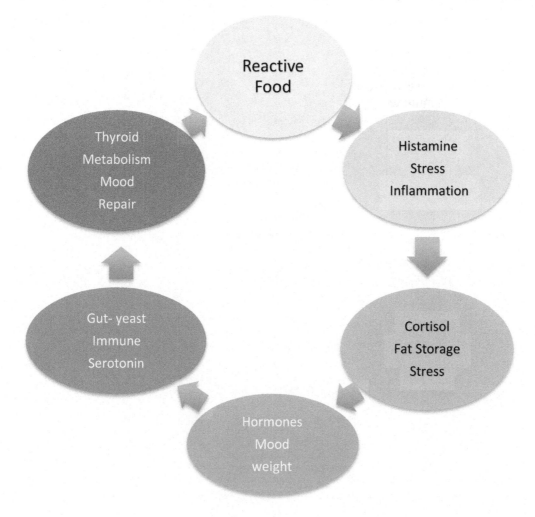

Here is a picture of what happens when you over exercise, especially over the age of 40

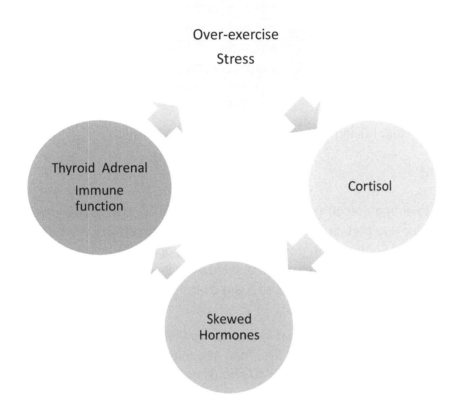

And the above diagram also shows what happens when you are stressed out. Now should be the aha/light blub moment. You are under constant stress!

Now it's time to fix it. Because all of these scenarios are affecting you in some way every day. Left unchecked what winds up happening is rampant weight gain and health issues.

When you identify and remove the factors that don't work for your body you can rapidly reverse this negative feedback loop.

Literally, in days, you can reset and restore your metabolism! Your body always wants to heal but it's always going to address whatever it thinks is a pressing problem. That pressing problem is stress.

I wrote The Metabolism Plan to help you identify all of the stimuli in your life that are causing you stress. When you hear that stress kills and stress makes you fat, it's not a myth. It's actual truth.

Heightened levels of cortisol affect your gut and immune function. This causes inflammation. Whenever you kick up inflammatory factors the effects can last for up to 72 hours. My goal, your goal, is to put you back in charge of your life by identifying and removing what doesn't work for you. From there we can make you healthier happier and leaner.

So let's get you back to having that metabolism of an 18-year-old!

Your Thyroid

When it comes to your metabolism your thyroid is the boss of you. Your thyroid is an important factor in every metabolic process in your body in fact every cell has receptors for thyroid hormones. So, if your thyroid is not operating optimally neither are you. This is why you want to find the food and exercise and lifestyle choices that support thyroid function. I don't want you don't fall into that "I am over 40 and it's normal to gain weight and feel like garbage" trap.

I know many of you I am sure have thyroid bloodwork that says that your thyroid is functioning optimally. My team and I at The Plan see this all the time. I can tell you 80% of the time this bloodwork is inaccurate. You should definitely resource The Metabolism Plan as to why on pages 23-27.

From a functional medicine point of view here's a diagram that explains why a traditional medical view might not see that you are functionally hypo or hyper thyroid.

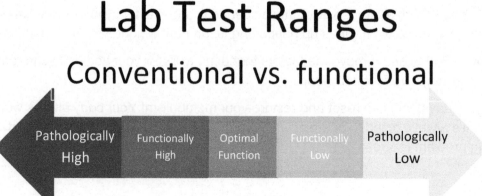

Lab Test Ranges
Conventional vs. functional

Pathologically High | Functionally High | Optimal Function | Functionally Low | Pathologically Low

Many doctors here in the US and abroad will only use TSH as a guideline which really doesn't mean that much if your T4 and T3 are low. You see T3 is really your metabolic powerhouse. You can have a decent level of TSH but still have a low level of T3. If T3 is low your metabolism is low.

Ok, this can obviously be a problem! What are some of the factors that can affect the conversion of TSH to T3?

This is the data that you will be observing in your Metabolism Plan Workbook. Hormones, sleep, exercise, stress and food are some of the major cofactors that will affect this conversion. Once you find the right formula for you it's back to being 110% with that teenage metabolism.

The Metabolism Plan is a wonderful journey, and you will be able to identify the factors that don't optimize your thyroid function. It all goes back to that concept that your body always wants to heal.

You will find that on the days that you over exercise your BBT – basal body temperature-will drop out of zone. You will find out when you get six hours asleep instead of 7 to 9 hours your bbt to drop. Well, what is BBT? Read on, because this is a huge part if your data gathering to repair your metabolism and having your best mood.

These are all things that you can fix and to me that's the most exciting thing about Planning. You collect YOUR data and then based on the data you make the best choices for your body.

Depression, Anxiety and Your BBT

What's really important about thyroid function is knowing that both depression and anxiety are tied to your thyroid. Often an underactive thyroid will result in depression, and an overactive thyroid will result in anxiety. But you can see you can see either condition with a dysfunctional thyroid.

And then there is gut function. 70 to 90% of serotonin your "I am happy" neurotransmitter is produced in your gut. When you are eating reactive foods your serotonin production and uptake is impaired.

As you restore and improve gut and thyroid function you will find, as many of my clients and staff have, that you are back to being a happier person! I can honestly say nothing makes me happier than hearing testimonials about how Planning has helped people with their depression.

CH , 35" I did the 30 days of the plan in May. I still have my one can of soda a day. I have my wine and chocolate every night. However, I found out that I am HIGHLY reactive to almonds, nuts, oatmeal, and multi-grain breads. All of which were staples in my vegetarian lactose intolerant diet. I have stayed away from those things. Not one has entered my mouth. Just from staying away from those things I am no longer on Prozac, which I had been on for 5 years for postpartum depression which never seemed to go away! I have been off Prozac for 4 months and my head just keeps getting clearer and clearer. My energy is more sustained. And I no longer have the anxiety and depression I lived with even while taking the medication. I was told I'd probably be on it the rest of my life."

So now that you're revved up to find out how to fix these problems naturally Let's go into some of the details

BBT

BBT stands for a basal body temperature, and you find out your BBT by taking an axillary temperature every morning. It's very simple, you just take a thermometer and put it under your armpit as soon as you wake up and then record that number. And I am going to say now, oral or forehead temps will not work!

A functional BBT is 96.5 to 96.9 and an optimal BBT is 97 to 97.3. When you fall out of the zones then there is thyroid impairment and The Metabolism Plan and this workbook is going to give you the tools to help fix it.

This method was developed by Dr. Broda Barnes a brilliant endocrinologist and researcher of thyroid function. He found that many people had "normal thyroid function" when looking at their bloodwork, when in fact they presented as being hypo or hyper thyroid. I have found this method of taking a daily BBT to be incredibly helpful for people suffering from a sluggish metabolism as well as for people that are on thyroid medications.

You may find that thyroid meds can be cut very quickly when observing identifying and removing the factors that are causing your metabolism to slow down. Of course, you should always check with your doctor. I highly suggest that people get their blood work done a few weeks after starting the Metabolism Plan to see if thyroid, and other medications, can be cut. Because it's just not thyroid meds. My team and I find that acid reflux medication, blood pressure medication, medication for type 2 diabetes, SSRIs, can often be titrated down. So please let your doctor know that you are starting a bio-individual anti-inflammatory diet so they can help monitor your progress.

LK- 43 "As a Family Practice physician I was never taught about nutrition or counseling patients regarding weight loss. Every day I am confronted with patient after patient describing their frustration and confusion over how to lose weight and I feel helpless. I try to guide them, but every person had different results, or no results, and as soon as they stopped rigidly following, they gained the weight back. I started to realize there was no one "diet" that fits everyone because we are all unique. That was when I read Lyn-Genet's article in a magazine and from a medical standpoint it made total sense, it is the missing component in nutrition science.

I recently tried to follow the calorie restriction and was confused that after 4 weeks I had only lost 3 lbs. Something had changed, my body had aged, and was not responding the same. I consulted Lyn-Genet who placed me on The Plan, within one week the 5 lbs were gone. I feel amazing, have more energy, have no acid reflux symptoms, no gastrointestinal issues (bloating), the 'sinus' headaches are gone as are the allergy pills. Best of all my clothes fit again, and I don't have to buy a new wardrobe! Figuring out what foods I react to and cutting them out of my diet has transformed my health and my body. This has been life changing experience and I will never look at food the same way.

I am thrilled to have another medical tool to help patients manage and eliminate their chronic condition such as migraines/arthritis/depression. For the first time I may be discontinuing medications instead of adding new ones."

Stress

Oh boy stress stress, stress!

It affects us all in so many ways and especially your health and your weight.

We tend to think of stress as just being something negative, but it can be a positive tool. Think of your first crush – that was a stress response, finding out you got a job promotion is a stress response that's pretty fun and that's pretty cool. But there are negative stressors and that's what we want to identify and learn how to manage.

Heightened levels of cortisol, without enough periods of rest from the stress is what really starts to affect our overall health and weight.

When you have more stress than your body can handle, your body goes into high alert. This heightened alert state is what starts a negative feedback loop

When you are constantly stressed you are preparing your body to always be in a state of fight or flight. You have to remember we have not biologically evolved that much since we were hunters and gatherers. When there were times of danger our bodies were always prepped for us to be ready to flee. Have you ever noticed that when you're stressed out you wake up at 3o'clock in the morning? That's a stress response.

Do you feel like you need to work out more and more to relieve the stress, but you're more and more stressed out? That's a stress response.

Are you having hot flashes all the time? I can almost bet you that you had a stressful day.

Stress will directly affect your thyroid. It decreases production of TSH and affects the conversion of T4 to T3.

Heightened levels of cortisol will usually decrease progesterone for women (it's known as progesterone steal) and in men will cut testosterone production. This is one of the reasons why we see so many mood disorders, because cortisol affects so many facets of your biology.

How Much Water YOU Need To Drink

The water guidelines are pretty basic, if you're outside the US convert your weight from kilos to pounds. Divide your weight number in pounds in half and that's how many ounces/liters of water you should drink.

Finish all of your water an hour before dinner if possible (45 minutes the latest) and finish all of your water by 7:30 at the latest.

Please don't have water with your meals as it can hamper digestion

Ex: if you weigh 160 pounds you will drink five 16 oz pints

1 pint at 7am

1 pint at 9am

1 pint at 11am

1 pint at 2pm

1 pint at 5pm

Tea will count towards your water up to 16 ounces, coffee soups and smoothies will not.

Black tea, peppermint tea, and chamomile tea are all approved after the cleanse. You can also have lemon juice in your water or lime juice in your water.

Sleep, Metabolism and Weight loss

So many of you think you can get by on six hours of sleep. But your bbt and your weight are saying something different. The less sleep you get the less weight you lose. In fact, for every two hours of sleep you don't get you can impact weight loss by up to a pound. So please, please do not get up early to exercise unless you get at least 7 hours of sleep!

You lose the most weight when your body is healing. That's why you can go to bed and why yourself and wake up the next day and be 2 pounds lighter. Your body is doing a deep repair and that requires a lot of energy.

So when you cut your sleep short to exercise, you're not only slowing weight loss. You're slowing deep healing. At the end of the day is the most important thing in the world. If you're 90 years old and you're dancing on the tabletops and 10 pounds heavier than your "goal weight", you're not going to care. Trust me, at the end of the day it's about being healthy and vital and happy and alive.

So, for all you folks that say, "Oh I can get by in five or six hours". I highly doubt it BUT measuring your BBT and weight every day is going to let you know exactly how much *your* body needs. So, if you get six hours instead of seven hours of sleep you might find that your weight stabilizes or you're up .2 to .4.

If you are consistently sleeping less than the minimum of seven hours you can be slowing down your long-term metabolism. You will know because your BBT will consistently drop.

Some days you will fall short of this goal. That's ok! You can't be perfect every day. But this workbook in conjunction with a Metabolism Plan is here to explain why that number is on the scale and why your metabolism may not be functioning as well as you like.

So, if you get six hours of sleep and your weight loss and BBT is impaired, is it going to kill you? No. The goal though is to understand how our body responds to our lifestyle choices and then to try to make it better.

What are some of the things that can impair our sleep? Stress of course is a big one. I can't tell you how many days I've woken up at 3 AM when I am stressed. Luckily, I have tools in my toolbelt that I am going to share with you!

1.Lemon Balm capsules are absolutely magic when you are having periods of disrupted sleep. As you lower stress levels and balance hormones you will find you need to use this less. I have seen people go from needing it nightly to just using it once or twice a week. Most people do well with 1500 mg 5-6 hours before bed. It gently unwinds you from the stress of the ay and it's also a great anxiety relief herb

2. Magnesium Cream – magnesium cream slathered on your feet at night can aid a SUPER deep sleep. I'm a huge fan of Cook's Organics. Magnesium helps you to relax (think an Epsom salt bath) and it's a wonderful part of your health tool kit.

3. Do not exercise after 5. Wait, huh?

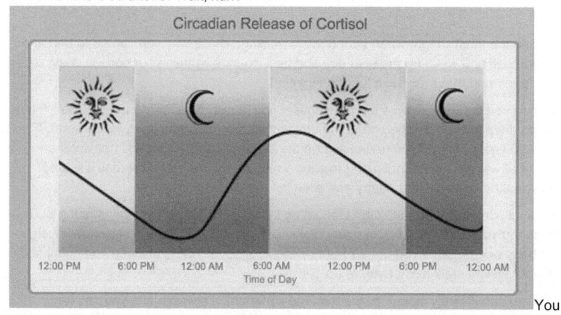

You have a natural peak that gets you up in the morning revved and ready to meet your day. You can see that it starts to really slow down by the time we hit 5 pm. This is our natural time to decompress from our busy life, relax, have a glass of wine or tea before dinner and then a nice nourishing dinner with friends and family.

When ones goes against this natural flow one can raise cortisol levels and one's body perceives this as danger, this translates to weight gain and metabolic slowdown.

If you find that your body is not responding optimally to your exercise choices you may want to rethink your after work gym visits. Try to get to bed earlier and do morning exercise!

For some people even baths and saunas after five can increase heart rate which your body can perceive as exertion and raise cortisol levels.

Does this mean you can't do it? Absolutely not! My job is never to say that this is good, or this is bad. My job is to help you get information that allows you to perceive your bio individual response to what you do in your life.

So if exercising or taking a hot bath or sauna after five works for you, I want you to do it. But if it stops working at some point, you can make different decisions.

I think it's really important to recognize that when you are less stressed you are going to pass more foods and exercise more. But when you are stressed, it's time for you to nourish yourself. Don't push so hard. Recognizing the ebb and flow in your life is really what The Metabolism Plan is all about.

Inflammation

Inflammation has been a hot buzzword and remains to be so because it really is the match to the wick for weight gain disease and premature aging.

Inflammation short term is great, that's what allows us to heal from a wound. But chronic low grade long-inflammation will start to affect gut function, the seat of your immune system.

But it's not just your health. It's also your mood. I discussed earlier that the majority of your "happy hormones" are also produced in your gut. Whatever supports your digestion is going to make you happy and strong and healthy. The exciting thing is when we support our best health and our best mood there will always be optimal weight... you don't need to diet. You just need to find what works for you.

Can't I Just Get a Food Sensitivity Test?

" We don't really understand all of the reasons why one person with anti-body response to a food will have serious reactions to the food, while another can eat it without problems. This is an area that needs more research," says Corinne A. Keet, associate professor of pediatrics at the Johns Hopkins University School of Medicine. To top it all off, it turns out that some studies show that an IgG response to a food actually indicates tolerance.

To make matters more confusing with blood tests? There has been research into the efficacy of blood tests. A few researchers had the same patient take a blood test in the morning and again in the afternoon and getting two very different results for their food sensitivities/allergies!

The European Academy of Allergy and Clinical Immunology stated that IgG tests should not be used to diagnose food sensitivities. The American Academy of Allergy, Asthma & Immunology then put out a statement noting that no serum antibody test, even the IgE tests that are sometimes helpful, can diagnose an allergy. They say flat-out: "The presence of antibody does not indicate disease." Plus, an antibody that doesn't show up on the test might be at undetectable levels, but that doesn't mean it's not there; you could still have an allergy to that food.

The Canadian Society of Allergy and Clinical Immunology weighed in saying positive test results for food-specific IgG are to be expected in normal, healthy adults and children. Furthermore, the inappropriate use of this test only increases the likelihood of false diagnoses being made, resulting in unnecessary dietary restrictions and decreased quality of life

Too often people come to me saying their blood test says they can't eat a food and when they test it on The Plan, they are fine. The most effective way to determine what food works for your chemistry is The Plan. You will find that your food sensitivities will change as you age, and that foods that you had to avoid you can now eat. The good news is that as your chemistry changes, the basic protocol of The Plan does not. You will always be able to determine what does, and doesn't work for you, using a very accurate and inexpensive methodology!

> ST- 49 *"I've paid tons of money for the ALCAT for my 18-year-old daughter who has Ankylosing Spondylitis. (3 different times!) and she never got results by avoiding the foods it said she reacted too.*
>
> *I told my daughter about your book and explained the commitment it would take from both of us to do it. I offered to do it along with her and we were buying vegetables I'd never heard of and using spices I'd never used before! It was an adjustment, but when you see the scale going down and your energy levels going up there's no stopping you. On day 5 I asked her if her pain was any better and she smiled at me and said, "I'm about a 4 now". That's amazing because on a scale of 1 -10 she was an 8 most of the time. This includes nighttime. She couldn't find relief sitting, standing, or lying down. I almost cried I was so happy for her.*
>
> *One day we were in a rush to get to my son's tournament, so we literally ran from the parking area. Suddenly my daughter shouted, "Mom, look at me, I'm running, and it doesn't hurt! We both laughed*

so hard. It was AWESOME and a memory I will never forget. Thank you so much for giving that to me and my daughter.

To sum it up, the ALCAT was way off. The Plan was dead on. I'm so grateful we are able to cancel her appointment with an RA doctor. She feels so blessed to have learned the proper way to eat at such a young age. Lyn-Genet, you have our eternal thanks!"

Auto immune disease

It is becoming widely accepted that putting autoimmune disease into remission is directly based on removing foods that cause leaky gut. These reactive foods, unique to your chemistry, are making you sick.

The results of Metabolism Planning, especially in conjunction with taking MSM for six weeks (see below) has helped people heal all over the world heal, eating foods they love without having to cut out entire food groups. There is no "bad" or good food, just what works for your body.

So what exactly is MSM?

MSM helps to alleviate the symptoms of many allergies including food allergies, contact allergies, seasonal allergies, etc. The major anti-allergic property of MSM is caused by its ability to bind to the mucosa and act as a "shield" between you and your allergens. MSM also helps to lower histamine levels.

By using MSM, reactive foods are deterred from entering the blood stream by this MSM shield and repairing your intestines. You can think of it as one big band-aid that allows your intestines to heal. This enables your body to repair and put AI into remission

Since an increase of MSM levels can stabilize your Ph balance, it helps to normalize stomach function and prevent overproduction of stomach acid. This also helps to alleviate heartburn and stomach ulcers.

What do I need to get started?

I'm not a big fan of supplements but I do believe in the short term that they can really help to maximize your health and act as a catalyst to your metabolism plan. Here's what you need for your first six weeks. See more about these supplements in the Tool Kit chapter.

- MSM is taken for six weeks (page 40)
- SAM-e only as needed for stress (page 41)
- Lemon balm only as needed (page 24)

- Probiotics only as needed (page 38)
- You will be taking your temperature for the first 30 days to gauge your response to exercise, sleep and stress, so please get a digital thermometer.
- Reliable scale, (withings.com)

In the beginning, there is a lot of cooking on the plan so if you have a crockpot, I highly recommend it. Chicken is an every other day protein - you can easily just put a crock of chicken in a crockpot with some carrots onions and fresh herbs and have the most delicious moist chicken in the world with no sodium and have several meals for the week. If you're a vegetarian make a big batch of lentils.

If there are other health issues that may require supplementation you can check out my website www.lyngenet.com for suggested brands.

The Cleanse Starts with NO Salt

This brings us to one of the biggest culprits with weight loss and with overall health. Too. Much. Salt.

Too much sodium causes water retention which not only affects our data but can raise blood pressure. The more salt we consume, the more we deaden our palate. So, we need more salt. In addition, studies have shown that too much sodium increases carbohydrate and sugar cravings. Great, so now you're puffy, bloated, and craving carbs. The quick fix? The Cleanse. Once or twice a year it is the perfect reset for your metabolism and health.

Now I don't want you to think that I am being negative about sodium! Sodium is an essential electrolyte for our bodies. But most of the food that you are ordering in, or the packaged food that you're eating, can contain 3 to 4 times amount of sodium we should be eating. Those convenience foods are anything less than convenient for your body.

Look at your labels and when you're eating out ask for no salt and salt it when it gets to the table if you need it.

Overview of Days 1 to 20

Days 1 to 3 - The cleanse

Days one through three are such an amazing time for allowing your body to reset and remove the factors that affect keeping you from being 100%.

Those healthy foods may be why your body is in a constant state of being reactive. This also means that you've probably been cutting out the "fun "foods because you are a motivated person.

Unfortunately, this scenario usually boils down to that you've been having less and less enjoyment eating foods that aren't working for your body (and are making you sick and fat).

That's just not really a way to live. I want you to break out of this cycle and incorporate more foods that make you happy and lower inflammation.

So, you start with The Cleanse which contains the least reactive foods. You start to build a foundation of foods that you love that work for your body. Easy, right?

In those first two weeks, I'm not going to let you start with a high reactive foods. So you salmon, turkey lovers and quinoa lovers I need you to hold off for a bit.

After the cleanse I want to introduce the foods that allow your body to rapidly heal. So, you might test halibut or flounder first and then if you pass that later you can test salmon.

But back to The Cleanse.

The first week we are testing foods which will allow you to build a foundation of foods that support your best weight and your best health. While these are all the least reactive foods, you may react to them. For instance, I have had people become reactive to almonds because they were eating them every day.

Expected weight loss during The Cleanse is anywhere from 5-7 lbs for a woman and 7-10 lbs for a man. If you lose less than a pound on day 1 when you test almonds for example, you are mildly reactive to almonds. Certainly, if you gain weight you are very reactive.

If you are mildly reactive to a food take a break and then retest it based on how much weight you gain.

Stabilization- retest in 3-6 months

Gain up to a lb- wait one year to retest.

Gain more than a lb wait 1 year plus.

Once you are at goal weight, stabilization is a pass. Women will have daily fluctuations of .2 or so. Men .4 or so.

The Cleanse Is Your Time to Heal

You may have done a detox before but many of the foods included in your detox may have been reactive.

When you eat foods that work for your body your body will rapidly release toxic build up which has been slowing your metabolism and affecting your health.

I don't want you to feel badly during the detox, but I do want you to eliminate many of the factors that could be keeping you from your best health.

For the first few days you can definitely take double strength peppermint tea which helps with nausea and headaches. I don't want you to have to suffer. This is not a draconian plan so, if you have a headache feel free to take an aspirin like Bayer or Excedrin migraine. I do find that and NSAIDs like Advil and Motrin will cause water retention. These will affect your weight loss.

You can watch days 1,2 and 3 on my YouTube channel – Lyn-Genet The Plan - for more tips.

As an omnivore are you going to introduce chicken at dinner and life becomes normal. As a vegetarian you're going to introduce lentils (the green-brown lentils are least reactive). They are both super strong proteins that can be eaten every other day. If you fail lentils, I suggest you try pinto beans as your next test.

These are the least reactive proteins that we start to work from, and we build a strong foundation from foods that nourish you, that your body loves and that you love to eat.

Days 4 to 10

You made it through Day 4 the cleanse, yay you! You're amazing.

Now life starts to get normal! You introduce coffee, wine, cheese, and chocolate on day four and this is where I am everyone's best friend.

We want to make sure to have a good mix of plant-based proteins to rotate so we start with one of life's great pleasure. Cheese.

Goat cheese is easier to digest than cow's cheese, so even if you have a dairy sensitivity, you will probably find you do great with a nice chevre or a sheep's cheese like manchego.

Some cow cheeses like Parmesan cheese are super low reactive but you can test that later.

If you find you are reactive to goat cheese, please go to my website-
www.lyngenet.com and download the failed goat cheese menu.

Day Five

You are going to test your first exercise!

6-8 minutes for beginners

10-12 minutes for intermediate

15 minutes for advanced

Now you may find that this baseline of time is all your body needs. You are looking for exercise to optimize weight loss. Keep track of your stats and see how you do!

Walking

Daily leisurely walks of 10 to 20 minutes are great. But walking, like anything else, may be perceived as stress.

Some people really can't exceed more than 7 to 8 thousand steps a day without stressing their bodies out (which you will note with a consistent dip of your bbt).

Others are like me where you need at least 10,000 steps to have your best metabolism. Will this data change over time? Absolutely, the more you lower stress levels the more stimulus your body can handle. So, if those hour-long hikes aren't working for you now, take a break. Let your body heal.

I would like you to start off with a baseline of 5000 steps a day and then slowly increase on your days when you're not exercising by 1000 steps a day That is approximately a 10-minute leisurely walk and let's see how you do.

Day Six

Time to test a new protein! Having at least three strong optimal proteins is essential for your Plan. Here is the optimal rotation of proteins if you pass them.

chicken 3x a week- every other day

lamb - 3x a week- every other day

eggs- 3 x a week every other day

beans- 3x a week- do not have more than once daily

duck breast- 3x a week every other day

fish and seafood - 2 x a week 3 days apart

vegetarian rice stir fry- 2x a week

pork- 1-2 x a week

turkey-1-2x a week

steak- 1x a week

bison- 1x every 5 days

buffalo- high reactive- please limit use if you pass

veal- high reactive- please limit use if you pass

Please choose from our lower reactive choices listed in your days 1-20. You can test higher reactive proteins like salmon and turkey after day 20.

Day Seven

I would like you to test a new exercise at the same baseline of time. So, if you tested an 8-minute run on day 5, test 8 minutes of weight training or Pilates on day 7.

BBT is not just an indicator of exercise which is why you can retest your exercise if it "fails". Sleep and stress are big factors in your BBT so don't be upset if your first exercise test does not go well.

So exactly what is optimal exercise? We're looking for an exercise to increase weight loss, optimize BBT, and lower body fat. If you find you have conflicting information or you were unclear the information, I hardly encourage you to retest the exercise at least three times.

Effective Exercise

1. You lose .6 or .8 instead of .4

2. Your bbt gets into a better zone

3. 3. You lose body fat (unless you are looking to bulk up). Here is an example of effective exercise with regards to body fat:

let's say your body fat is 20%

Effective exercise
1st day post exercise 19.2% body fat
2nd day post exercise 19% body fat

Not optimal exercise
1st day post 20.4% body fat
2nd day post exercise 20% body fat

Lousy exercise
1st day post exercise 21% body fat
2nd day post exercise 20.4% body fat

It's also important for everyone to have 2 to 3 types of exercise that support their body. So, if you're a runner perhaps investigate weight training and yoga.

If you're a bodybuilder definitely look into yoga and Pilates.

Day Eight

You are building your food foundation, so you need more proteins to rotate.

Once you pass three strong optimal proteins then you get to the next phase which is testing a new vegetable. Please do not move forward to a new test until you pass previous tests.

Day Nine

You have more choices now!

1. Increase an approved exercise by 20%

2. Test a new exercise

3. Retest an exercise.

So, if you think you "failed" 10 minute of yoga, but you love it, please retest at least 3 times.

What happens if you still fail yoga? Well, maybe you were doing yoga too often and your body needs a break. Don't fret, it will come back into your regimen when your body is ready for it.

Rotate or React is a strong principle with Planning and that means exercise too. Maybe try running and yoga in summer and weight training and Pilates in winter. Your body always does best with new stimulus every 6 months or so. That's also why eating seasonally is so effective too!

Day 10

Protein is essential for repair, and your body loses the most weight (and you are your healthiest) when it's repairing. Because we need to rotate our foods, I want you to be able to rotate your dinner proteins as much as possible. At this point I hope you have found three proteins besides chicken or lentils that suit your body

Of course, if you look at the Rotate or React principal, you may see that you might have failed some proteins if you've been overeating them. For instance, if you've been eating fish 3 to 4 times a week you may find that it fails.

Do not be stressed out by "failing". It's actually your body being incredibly wise and saying, "Hey, I need a break." The best thing you can do is listen! Definitely watch my Rotate or React videos on YouTube. I can promise you I develop this protocol and I have failed everything by not listening to my own rules LOL. I have lost chicken, fish, cheese, pumpkin seeds…you name it.

Let's face it, we're all creatures of habit. I fall victim to the same issues as you, but we can all try to do better. It's also really exciting to know that when you identify a food that's causing inflammation, you can keep it out of your diet for a while and re-introduce it.

Days 11 and beyond

This is the basic premise you are going to follow for days 11-20. Even numbered days test a new food. Odd-numbered days test a new exercise or stay with approved exercise.

Remember you can't move onto a new test until you pass previous tests.

If you have passed 3 proteins

Day 12- test a new vegetable- suggestions are potato, fennel, snow peas or spinach

Day 13- test increased exercise by 20% or test a new exercise

Day 14- test bread if you passed the vegetable test. If not, test a new vegetable

Day 15- test exercise

Day 16- test a new snack such as pecans or test wild rice for a new lunch protein

Day 17- test exercise

Day 18- test a restaurant or test a new fruit- suggestions mango, raspberries, or pomegranate and in summer apricot or nectarine

Day 19- test a new exercise and start working on days 21-25 with your self menu template (**www.lyngenet.com**)

Day 20- repeat your best day and pat yourself on the back!

There is more guidance on YouTube for each day if you need it.

Days 21-30 you will start to make your own menus

Until day 30 you will test foods on the even numbered days, building an arsenal of foods that work for your chemistry. On the odd numbered days you will test exercise finding out what works to make you strong and lean, without stressing your metabolism and adrenals out.

If you have been overexercising, you may find you need to rein it in a little and let your body geal.

If you haven't been exercising because you thought you needed to exercise an hour a day 5-6 days a week you are in for a wonderful surprise! You may just need to exercise 8-12 minutes every other day.

Don't forget your "off exercise". That means leisurely walks or gentle yoga and abs, that get you moving without stressing your body out.

Planning is all about listening to our body, When you do that you will always win.

Meantime, I hope you enjoyed this companion workbook to my two books The Plan and The Metabolism Plan.

Introduction to The Plan

Preparation

You will need:

- A digital scale, which measures in 2/10th of a pound. I prefer *Withings* (withings.com). Eatsmart is no longer working as well. I just threw mine out the window!

- A digital thermometer

- MSM

- SAM-e or Lemon Balm for stress

- Probiotic

Please HYDRATE! Your baseline is half your body weight in ounces - the best way to do this is drink a pint all at once. Please drink water in-between meals, not during as drinking during meals can impair your digestion--If you can leave a 45 window before and after each meal that is ideal.

Do *not drink any water (yes that means tea too!) after dinner* and try to finish all water by 7:30 or 3-4 hours before bed. Please do not drink over the recommended water amount as this may stress kidney function and will cause slow weight loss.

General Guidelines

- Please follow the menus exactly. Do not make substitutions or changes without prior approval.

- Do not swap lunch and dinner from different days. Ex: day 5 lunch with day 4 dinner.

- Please start each day with 16 oz of water and fresh lemon juice plus MSM for 6 weeks.

Many clients ask about eating out and we discourage this in the first few weeks because too much of weight gain comes from excess sodium and a meal prepared in a restaurant can have 3 days' worth of sodium! This is why we ask that you please wait until day 18 to dine out.

Do not work out the first four days. This is detox time when the body is repairing your organs. If you work out during this time, energy is spent on muscle repair instead of repairing vital organs. You have the rest of your life to work out. RELAX! You can do leisurely walks, with no elevated heart rate for up to 20 minutes.

- If you feel tired, this is an indication that the body has a lot of repair to do and listen to it! Your body is getting a break from digesting reactive foods and wants to repair.

- Use only lemon juice and extra-virgin olive oil for salad dressing, unless otherwise indicated.

- No vinegar until Day 4.

- No coffee until after Day 4 (If you think you are going to get a headache, drink black tea with coconut milk— up to 2 cups).

- If you drink two fewer glasses of your recommended daily water intake, you may retain .5 lbs of water weight.

Do NOT "overload" your body at the end of the day to make up what you didn't drink earlier. This can overload your kidneys and will most likely show up as water retention the next morning. Please drink your last pint of water an hour before your dinner. If you drink water after dinner, it will hamper digestion and show up as weight gain.

The lower your weight, the less water intake you require.

Hurray!

So the calculation is your body weight in pounds divided in half.

Reactions

When you are reactive to a food, it can take up to 72 hours for normal functioning to resume. This will include weight loss, normal bowel movements, return of digestive functioning, and a decrease in your genetic "maladies." Taking a probiotic after a reactive food will help you regain normal functioning sooner.

Probiotics

Please only take a probiotic on an as needed basis. You want your biome to be as diverse as possible. Taking the same strains every day will actually lessen diversity, especially if the strains you are taking are already dominant! When getting a probiotic please watch out for prebiotics as they maty increase digestive issues, fermentation and yeast. I like Renew Life 30 billion or Innate.

Coffee

- After Day 3 you may drink 1 cup of coffee per day with half and half or coconut milk. You can also mix water with cream if half and half is not available. Your choice of sweeteners are honey and agave. If you don't have those then brown or white sugar is fine. maple syrup, and yes – plain old sugar.   Do not have any other sweetener including stevia.

Salt

- No salt until after Day 4. After Day 4, sea salt may be used in moderation. You will find that after the cleanse, your taste for salt will have decreased significantly. Pink Himalayan is my fave! If you are an avid exerciser (over 75 minutes per day), you may need over the 1500-1800 mg referenced in The Metabolism Plan. Remember all food contains naturally occurring sodium too so you may need less depending on what you eat.

General Food Guidelines

- Chicken – thighs beasts, drumsticks – I don't care. Eat what makes you happy. Portion size for women is 4-6 oz. Portion size for men is 6-8 oz. You can test larger portion sizes later in your plan, especially if you increase exercise.

- Nuts — Choose only raw, unsalted nuts. Roasted nuts are 95% reactive. Men should have 1.5 - 2 oz as their serving (a large handful), women should have 1 oz (a large handful).

Oils

- Cooking at high temperatures can damage oils. The more Omega-3 fatty acids in the oil, the less suitable it is for cooking. Heat not only damages the fatty acids, it can also change them into harmful substances. Olive oil and avocado oil are best for cooking as long as you do not heat it above its smoke point. 350°F (175°C) for olive oil, 500° F for avocado. Avocado oil is great for baking.

Wine

- Wine is WONDERFUL in moderation. It enhances digestion, is a mild diuretic and decreases stress. One glass of red wine is allowed beginning on Day 4. Do not consume white wine as it is more acidic and will slow weight loss. Wine is allowed with or after dinner as it aids digestion and decreases cortisol.

Your Tool Kit

Methylsulfonylmethane (MSM)

MSM and Allergies

MSM helps to alleviate the symptoms of a large number of allergies including food allergies, contact allergies, inhalation allergies, etc. The major anti-allergic property of MSM is caused by its ability to bind to the mucosa and present a natural blocking interface between hosts and allergens.

What do we use MSM for at The Plan?
- Acid Reflux
- Allergies- food and environmental
- Arthritis
- Asthma
- Healthy collagen synthesis - skin, hair, nails and joints
- Inflammation (especially of mucous membranes)
- Leaky gut

MSM is my everything and you will soon find out why. When I first started people on it, I only used it for reducing histamine and seasonal allergies. Soon I found it did much, much more.

You can see how it impacted my life on my YouTube video and how it has helped so many people recover form GERD, asthma, autoimmune disease, chronic pain and even depression!

How do I take MSM?

Therapeutic dosage is 3,000-6,000 mg and long-term change has been seen after 6 weeks of usage. Dosage is based on weight.

Weight	Daily MSM Dosage
100 to 180 lb	3,000 mg
180 to 240 lb	4,000 mg
240+ lb	5,000 mg

SAM-e

What do we use SAM-e for at The Plan?

Stress, or heightened levels of cortisol, enact long term fat storage which leads to weight gain. In addition, stress disrupts hormonal balance and attacks our master gland for our metabolism, the thyroid. Thyroid dysfunction is linked to depression and anxiety disorders. Thyroid dysfunction affects at least 30 million Americans, with many more undiagnosed to their condition. Mitigating the effects of stress is crucial for optimal weight loss and metabolic function

Cortisol exacerbates our tendency to store visceral fat, the fat around our abdomen. The fat cells that lie in the abdomen have been linked to increased rates of diabetes which affects 30 million Americans with 86 million with pre-diabetes. Visceral fat has also been linked to increased risk of heart disease which affects 47% of the US.

At The Plan we have found SAM-e's unique effects to lower response to stress enhance weight loss and overall health. When combined with MSM and probiotics to strengthen digestion and the microbiome, traditional weight loss models are obsolete.

SAM-e stands for S-adenosyl methionine and is made in the body from a reaction between methionine, an amino acid and adenosine triphosphate. SAMe- is involved in many different reactions in the body and levels drop as we age. It is used to treat depression, stress, liver problems, fibromyalgia, musculoskeletal pain and arthritis. It is also used to treat cognitive decline and Alzheimer's. Many women use SAM-e for hormonal problems including PMS and PMDD. It has been shown to increase serotonin.

SAMe is the most active of all methyl donors and has been compared to ATP in its importance for the body. SAMe is involved in the synthesis of:

• Neurotransmitters

• The hormone melatonin

• Phospholipids

• Polyamines, which control cellular growth

It is also the source of methyl groups inside the nucleus for DNA methylation, which controls gene expression and masking of genetic damage.

SAMe was shown to improve liver function and provide protection from the hepatotoxic effects of medications (i.e., acetaminophen), alcohol, and other toxins. It increases synthesis of glutathione, and it is a precursor of taurine and phosphatidylcholine, which are essential in detoxification pathways. These functions of SAMe could potentially be helpful for women taking HRT or BCPs, and those suffering from cholestasis and heavy metal toxicity.

SAMe was found very helpful in preventing and reversing the damage caused by both osteo and rheumatoid arthritis through the following mechanisms:

• Regeneration of the joint tissues by increasing the number of chondrocyte cells which are responsible for the production of the collagen matrix, proteoglycans and chondroitin sulfate

• Counteracts the destructive effect of the inflammatory cytokine TNF-alpha

Allowing for the synthesis of chondroitin sulfate via supplementation of SAMe may make more sense than trying to supplement chondroitin sulfate, which is a large and difficult to absorb molecule. Many of the quality studies supporting the use of chondroitin sulfate were conducted with intravenous administration.

In addition, by improving serotonin levels, SAMe might improve pain tolerance in patients with fibromyalgia and other pain disorders.

Lemon Balm- Lemon balm is a natural anti-anxiety herb which supports a healthy mood, focus, optimal sleep and a feeling of well-being. Most people with sleep issues do well with 1500 mg taken 5-6 hours before bed.

Frequently Asked Questions - General

Should I stop my medications when I start The Plan?

While we do often find that medications can be cut down dramatically once you get started, please make sure to discuss with your doctor before you discontinue or taper down any medication. Bloodwork is recommended 30 days after starting the plan to review medications with your doctor.

Can I do The Plan if I'm breastfeeding?

For moms still breastfeeding, The Plan works beautifully, but should only be done under the care of one of our staff because the weight loss on The Plan is very rapid and we may need to adjust variables so that it does affect breast milk supply.

I'm under 35, can I still do The Plan?

Yes! Doing The Plan under age 35 is still very valuable to improve health. For clients that are under 35 and have a chronic health condition (eczema, migraines, diabetes, etc.) weight is still a very accurate gauge. However, we have found that weight is not as accurate of a gauge of reactivity for those under 35 who don't have a chronic health condition, we recommend paying attention to the physical cues (gas/bloating, constipation/diarrhea, headaches, fatigue) as indications to discovering your reactive foods.

I'm doing The Plan for health reasons, but don't want to lose any more weight?

We work with many clients who want to improve their health but do not need to lose weight. We have found that during the cleanse you may still lose a small amount of weight as the body lets go of inflammation, but the body will quickly find its natural set point where weight will stabilize. At this point, you can judge reactivity by seeing weight go up and a friendly day will be where the weight stays at your set point.

I'm concerned that I have a health issue that would prevent me from doing The Plan. How do I find out?

The Plan can work for everybody (that's the beauty of a program that's about *your* individual chemistry!). However, there are some conditions, such as diverticulitis or ulcerative colitis where we do prefer that you work directly with one of our highly trained staff to create a custom menu based on your current diet. If you aren't sure what is best in your particular situation, please email info@lyngenet.com to inquire.

How does a woman's monthly cycle impact testing and reactivity?

Many women find that their weight stabilizes/goes up and their reactive response is amplified the 2-3 days prior to their cycle because of hormone-related water retention.

Let's say a food, i.e.: fish is really only mildly reactive to you and normally cause you to stabilize, if you're PMSing, it can amplify that reactive response a .5 - 1 lb. gain. Every woman is different with the amount of gain they see and for how long, so make sure to pay attention to your cycles before you start The Plan to have a sense of how your body typically responds! As you continue The Plan, hormone balance dramatically improves, so every month you are on The Plan, you will see less water retention and fewer PMS symptoms prior to your cycle.

A good rule of thumb for most women is to avoid testing new foods (stick with friendly days) 2-3 days prior to your cycle. Once you start your cycle and feel good, you can pick right back up with testing and collecting your data.

This is a great time to test more exercise which will optimize bbt and hormones and help with the PMS.

I am worried that I might be hungry, especially during the cleanse?

Not at all! In fact, we often have clients who can't finish every meal. Each meal is chemically balanced, and you eat until you are full. In fact, as a woman you are consuming 2000 calories, as a man over 2800 and the cleanse is rich with protein, fat and fiber.

Is there an alternative to the Flax Granola?

Until you test more foods, you can substitute the Blueberry Pear Compote or the smoothie. It will not have the exact same digestive benefits as the flax and some people find it less filling. The recipe can be found in our menus.

Water Questions

Why can't you drink with meals?

Drinking water with meals dilutes digestive enzymes, which will impair digestion. It also causes you to be prematurely full and we want you to fill up on food so that you aren't hungry in an hour or two! It is best to wait 45 minutes before and after your meals to have water.

Does coffee count as part of my water intake when I include it starting on day 4?

Coffee does not count towards your daily water total.

Should I add extra water for wine and when is it best to have wine?

Yes! It's best to add an extra 4-5 oz. to your daily total for every glass of wine you have and it's good to include that water earlier in the day (before 7:30 pm). You can have wine later at night (up until bedtime!).

What can I do if I am drinking all my water but am still thirsty?

I would first make sure that you added in any extra water that you might need for wine or exercise. If you are still thirsty at this point, then please try adding lemon juice to your water. The extra vitamin C helps the cells of the body to absorb and use the water more efficiently, so you will feel less thirsty.

How do I adjust my water intake for exercise?

A good rule of thumb is to add in 8 oz. for every 30 minutes of exercise. You may drink less or more according to thirst. Keep exercise to 20 minutes the first 10-14 days for best results. Intense exercise may slow weight loss.

How do I adjust water intake for hot weather?

In hot weather, make adjustments similar to exercise (one or two additional glasses depending upon the severity of the heat, how much time you spend outdoors, etc.). This is especially important for those of you who get migraines because heat can dehydrate you and trigger migraines. Staying out in the heat too long can start to cause your body to overheat and impair your lymphatic system. We see this especially when gardening outdoors for hours. It is best to take breaks from the heat by going inside and cooling off every 30 minutes if possible. You may notice weight stabilization in the next day.

Days 1-20 Menu

Day One

Plan Menu for Day	What you actually ate:
Breakfast • 1 cup Flax granola with ½ cup blueberries • Silk Coconut milk or Rice Dream- these will be your breakfast "milk" for the week.	
Lunch • 16oz of Carrot ginger soup • 2 cups of sautéed or steamed broccoli drizzle with orange oil and lemon juice • Baby Romaine with 1 oz sunflower seeds	
Snack - 1 Apple	
Dinner • Sautéed kale, 3-4 carrots, onion, zucchini, shiitakes, and broccoli with spicy coco sauce with a handful of sunflower seeds • Grated Carrot and raw grated beet salad with a handful of pumpkin seeds *When you make the spicy coco sauce: make the sauce, add all the vegetables to it and let it simmer for 10 minutes*	
Results	
Date:	
Supplements and medications on or recommended:	
Plan Day Followed yesterday:	
Any menu deviations yesterday:	
Water consumed (ounces) yesterday:	
Hours Slept yesterday:	
Exercise yesterday:	
Weight (pounds) today:	
BBT (F) today:	
Digestion yesterday and this morning:	
Mood yesterday and this morning:	
Stress Level yesterday and this morning:	

Day Two: Almonds

Plan Menu for Day	What you actually ate:
Breakfast • 1 cup of Flax with ½ cup blueberries.	
Lunch • 16oz of Carrot ginger soup with 1 oz of sunflower seeds • Baby romaine with ½ diced apple, ¼ avocado • 2 cups of steamed or sautéed broccoli	
Snack - 1 pear with 8 almonds	
Dinner • Leftover sautéed kale and veggies with 1 cup basmati rice with pumpkin seeds beet/carrot salad with and handful of sunflower seeds	
Results	
Date:	
Supplements and medications on or recommended:	
Plan Day Followed yesterday:	
Any menu deviations yesterday:	
Water consumed (ounces) yesterday:	
Hours Slept yesterday:	
Exercise yesterday:	
Weight (pounds) today:	
BBT (F) today:	
Digestion yesterday and this morning:	
Mood yesterday and this morning:	
Stress Level yesterday and this morning:	

Day Three: Chicken

Plan Menu for Day	What you actually ate:
Breakfast • 1 cup Flax with choice of ½ cup blueberries or ½ pear	
Lunch • Baby romaine with carrots and a handful of sunflower seeds • 16oz of Cream of Broccoli soup	
Snack - 12-15 almonds	
Dinner • ½ portion chicken (2-3 oz) with Italian herbs and orange zest on a bed of baby romaine • Oven roasted zucchini, broccoli, carrots, onions, garlic and Italian herb blend	

Results	
Date:	
Supplements and medications on or recommended:	
Plan Day Followed yesterday:	
Any menu deviations yesterday:	
Water consumed (ounces) yesterday:	
Hours Slept yesterday:	
Exercise yesterday:	
Weight (pounds) today:	
BBT (F) today:	
Digestion yesterday and this morning:	
Mood yesterday and this morning:	
Stress Level yesterday and this morning:	

Day Four: Cheese

(You may now have one cup of coffee in the morning and wine at   night with or after dinner)

Plan Menu for Day	What you actually ate:
Breakfast • 1 cup flax Granola with ½ cup berries, ½ apple or ½ pear.	
Lunch • Leftover reheated, roasted vegetables on a bed of baby romaine with and handful of pumpkin seeds and 1oz of goat cheese	
Snack – • Carrots with 2 Tbsp raw almond butter Or • Plan Trail Mix ⅛ cup sunflower and ⅛ cup craisins	
Dinner • 4-6oz of Chicken with lemon, garlic, and rosemary • Baby Romaine or frisée with carrots and ¼ avocado • Steamed or sautéed broccoli with yellow squash, lemon and dill	
Results	
Date:	
Supplements and medications on or recommended:	
Plan Day Followed yesterday:	
Any menu deviations yesterday:	
Water consumed (ounces) yesterday:	
Hours Slept yesterday:	
Exercise yesterday:	
Weight (pounds) today:	
BBT (F) today:	
Digestion yesterday and this morning:	
Mood yesterday and this morning:	
Stress Level yesterday and this morning:	

Day Five: Test Exercise

beginner 4-6 min ~ intermediate/adv 10-12 min

Plan Menu for Day	What you actually ate:
Breakfast • The Plan Smoothie. •	
Lunch • Green leaf lettuce with radicchio, carrot/beet salad and handful of sunflower seeds 16oz of Cream of Broccoli soup	
Snack – • Carrots with 2 Tbsp raw almond butter Or ½ apple with raw almond butter	
Dinner • 4-6oz of Chicken with spicy apricot glaze on a bed of green leaf • Sautéed zucchini, yellow squash with onion or leeks and basil finish with lemon and ½ oz manchego	

Results	
Date:	
Supplements and medications on or recommended:	
Plan Day Followed yesterday:	
Any menu deviations yesterday:	
Water consumed (ounces) yesterday:	
Hours Slept yesterday:	
Exercise yesterday:	
Weight (pounds) today:	
BBT (F) today:	
Digestion yesterday and this morning:	
Mood yesterday and this morning:	
Stress Level yesterday and this morning:	

Day Six: Protein Day

Plan Menu for Day	What you actually ate:
Breakfast • Blueberry Compote	
Lunch • Baby romaine with wilted radicchio, ¼ avocado, handful of pumpkin seeds and 1oz of goat cheese • Lemon basil escarole soup	
Snack • ½ apple and raw almond butter Or • Carrots and zucchini noush- 2 Tbsp	
Dinner: – *choose your proteins to test* • 4-6oz of wild halibut or flounder, steak, lamb, duck or 3 eggs with 2 cups kale • Grilled vegetables- zucchini, yellow squash, carrots, onion, radicchio • Carrot beet salad with sunflower seeds	

Results	
Date:	
Supplements and medications on or recommended:	
Plan Day Followed yesterday:	
Any menu deviations yesterday:	
Water consumed (ounces) yesterday:	
Hours Slept yesterday:	
Exercise yesterday:	
Weight (pounds) today:	
BBT (F) today:	
Digestion yesterday and this morning:	
Mood yesterday and this morning:	
Stress Level yesterday and this morning:	

Day Seven: Test Exercise

beginner 4-6 min – intermediate/adv 10-12 min

Plan Menu for Day	What you actually ate:
Breakfast • Flax Granola with ½ cup berries, ½ apple or ½ pear Or • Apple Streusel	
Lunch • Leftover vegetables on a bed of green leaf with handful of sunflower seeds • Chicken Kale Soup	
Snack – • 1 oz salt free potato chips Or • Carrots and Zucchini-noush – 2 Tbsp	
Dinner • Chicken with dill and lemon • Sautéed vegetables- broccoli, carrots, zucchini, with garlic • Frisée or baby romaine salad	
Results	
Date:	
Supplements and medications on or recommended:	
Plan Day Followed yesterday:	
Any menu deviations yesterday:	
Water consumed (ounces) yesterday:	
Hours Slept yesterday:	
Exercise yesterday:	
Weight (pounds) today:	
BBT (F) today:	
Digestion yesterday and this morning:	
Mood yesterday and this morning:	
Stress Level yesterday and this morning:	

Day Eight: Test New protein

Plan Menu for Day	What you actually ate:
Breakfast • The Plan Smoothie.	
Lunch • Leftover sautéed vegetables (½ cup broccoli) on a bed of green leaf with 1oz of goat cheese and handful of sunflower seeds • basil escarole soup	
Snack – • Carrots with 2 Tbsp raw almond butter Or • Pumpkin seeds	
Dinner • Test 4-6oz of a new protein on a bed of green leaf or frisée • Roasted, Sautéed, Grilled or steamed vegetables that have been approved	
Results	
Date:	
Supplements and medications on or recommended:	
Plan Day Followed yesterday:	
Any menu deviations yesterday:	
Water consumed (ounces) yesterday:	
Hours Slept yesterday:	
Exercise yesterday:	
Weight (pounds) today:	
BBT (F) today:	
Digestion yesterday and this morning:	
Mood yesterday and this morning:	
Stress Level yesterday and this morning:	

Day Nine: Test Exercise

beginner 4-6 min~ intermediate 10-12 min ~ advanced 15 min

Plan Menu for Day	What you actually ate:
<u>Breakfast</u> • Apple Streusel Or • Blueberry pear compote	
<u>Lunch</u> • Baby Romaine with ¼ avocado and grated carrots • 1.5 cups Roasted broccoli with 1 oz manchego (heated up)	
<u>Snack</u> • Pumpkin seeds Or • Plan Trail Mix	
<u>Dinner</u> • Chicken • Baby Romaine with grated raw beet • Sautéed zucchini or yellow squash, carrots and leeks	

Results	
Date:	
Supplements and medications on or recommended:	
Plan Day Followed yesterday:	
Any menu deviations yesterday:	
Water consumed (ounces) yesterday:	
Hours Slept yesterday:	
Exercise yesterday:	
Weight (pounds) today:	
BBT (F) today:	
Digestion yesterday and this morning:	
Mood yesterday and this morning:	
Stress Level yesterday and this morning:	

Day Ten: Test new protein

Plan Menu for Day	What you actually ate:
Breakfast • Flax Granola with ½ pear or blueberries Or • Blueberry pear compote	
Lunch • Chicken Kale soup • Red leaf or Green leaf lettuce with carrot/beet salad with sunflower seeds	
Snack – • Pumpkin seeds Or • ½ apple with raw almond butter	
Dinner • Test New Protein • Sautéed kale with onion, basil and fresh lime • Any lettuce used thus far with ¼ avocado and fresh herbs such as dill, basil or mint	
Results	
Date:	
Supplements and medications on or recommended:	
Plan Day Followed yesterday:	
Any menu deviations yesterday:	
Water consumed (ounces) yesterday:	
Hours Slept yesterday:	
Exercise yesterday:	
Weight (pounds) today:	
BBT (F) today:	
Digestion yesterday and this morning:	
Mood yesterday and this morning:	
Stress Level yesterday and this morning:	

Day Eleven: Test increased exercise time by 20%

Plan Menu for Day	What you actually ate:
Breakfast • Blueberry Pear Compote Or Smoothie.	
Lunch • Lettuce of choice with grated carrot, ¼ avocado, sunflower seeds and dried cranberries • Chicken Kale Soup	
Snack – • Carrots with raw almond butter Or • ½ apple with raw almond butter	
Dinner • Any approved protein • 1 cup Vegetable timbale and 1 cup sautéed zucchini • Any lettuce used thus far with fresh herbs	

Results	
Date:	
Supplements and medications on or recommended:	
Plan Day Followed yesterday:	
Any menu deviations yesterday:	
Water consumed (ounces) yesterday:	
Hours Slept yesterday:	
Exercise yesterday:	
Weight (pounds) today:	
BBT (F) today:	
Digestion yesterday and this morning:	
Mood yesterday and this morning:	
Stress Level yesterday and this morning:	

Day Twelve: Test new vegetable

Plan Menu for Day	What you actually ate:
Breakfast • The Plan Smoothie Or • Blueberry pear Compote.	
Lunch • 1.5 cups Roasted Broccoli with Plan Caesar • Salad with ¼ avocado and sunflower seeds	
Snack • Carrots and zucchini noush (2 Tbsp) Or • Carrots and raw almond butter	
Dinner • Approved protein • Test new vegetable mixed with other approved vegetables- use herbs of choice • Any lettuce used thus far with fresh herbs and raw grated beet	
Results	
Date:	
Supplements and medications on or recommended:	
Plan Day Followed yesterday:	
Any menu deviations yesterday:	
Water consumed (ounces) yesterday:	
Hours Slept yesterday:	
Exercise yesterday:	
Weight (pounds) today:	
BBT (F) today:	
Digestion yesterday and this morning:	
Mood yesterday and this morning:	
Stress Level yesterday and this morning:	

Day Thirteen: Test increased exercise time by 20%

Plan Menu for Day	What you actually ate:
Breakfast • Flax granola with ½ cup approved fruit	
Lunch • Leftover vegetables with sunflower seeds, ¼ chopped apple on a bed of green leaf lettuce • Chicken Kale Soup	
Snack • Pumpkin seeds Or • Low Sodium Potato Chips	
Dinner • Approved protein • Any lettuce used thus far with fresh herbs and optional radicchio • 1 cup vegetable timbale- sautéed zucchini noodles •	
Results	
Date:	
Supplements and medications on or recommended:	
Plan Day Followed yesterday:	
Any menu deviations yesterday:	
Water consumed (ounces) yesterday:	
Hours Slept yesterday:	
Exercise yesterday:	
Weight (pounds) today:	
BBT (F) today:	
Digestion yesterday and this morning:	
Mood yesterday and this morning:	
Stress Level yesterday and this morning:	

Day Fourteen: Optional test bread

Plan Menu for Day	What you actually ate:
Breakfast • Any approved breakfast Or • Test Bread with raw almond butter and ½ piece of fruit	
Lunch • Basil escarole soup -optional • Salad with 15 grams of vegetarian protein Example of hitting protein goals: ○ 1.5 oz of goat cheese and sunflower seeds ○ 2 cups sautéed kale and 1 oz pumpkin seeds ○ 2 cups cream of broccoli soup and 1oz almond slivers ○ 2 cups chicken kale soup and 1 cup broccoli	
Snack - Carrots and Zucchini-noush (2 Tbsp) Or ½ apple	
Dinner • Approved protein • Roasted, Sautéed or Grilled Vegetables that have been approved • Any approved lettuce with fresh herbs	
Results	
Date:	
Supplements and medications on or recommended:	
Plan Day Followed yesterday:	
Any menu deviations yesterday:	
Water consumed (ounces) yesterday:	
Hours Slept yesterday:	
Exercise yesterday:	
Weight (pounds) today:	
BBT (F) today:	
Digestion yesterday and this morning:	
Mood yesterday and this morning:	
Stress Level yesterday and this morning:	

Day Fifteen: Test increased exercise time by 20%

Plan Menu for Day	What you actually ate:
Breakfast • Flax Granola with ½ piece of apple or ½ pear	
Lunch • Carrot Ginger soup- optional • Salad with 15 grams of vegetarian protein	
Snack • Low Sodium Potato chips Or • ½ cup blueberries	
Dinner • Chicken with spices of choice • Sautéed kale with onions and zucchini and new approved vegetable • Any approved lettuce with fresh herbs	

Results	
Date:	
Supplements and medications on or recommended:	
Plan Day Followed yesterday:	
Any menu deviations yesterday:	
Water consumed (ounces) yesterday:	
Hours Slept yesterday:	
Exercise yesterday:	
Weight (pounds) today:	
BBT (F) today:	
Digestion yesterday and this morning:	
Mood yesterday and this morning:	
Stress Level yesterday and this morning:	

Day Sixteen: Test new snack

Plan Menu for Day	What you actually ate:
Breakfast • Blueberry Pear Compote Or • Streusel	
Lunch • Basil escarole soup • Salad with 15 grams of vegetarian protein	
Snack • Test 1oz Pecans Or • Test new fruit- ½ portion (ex: ½ cup mango or blackberries)	
Dinner • Approved protein • Steamed, Grilled or sautéed approved vegetables • Any approved lettuce with fresh herbs and grated carrots	

Results	
Date:	
Supplements and medications on or recommended:	
Plan Day Followed yesterday:	
Any menu deviations yesterday:	
Water consumed (ounces) yesterday:	
Hours Slept yesterday:	
Exercise yesterday:	
Weight (pounds) today:	
BBT (F) today:	
Digestion yesterday and this morning:	
Mood yesterday and this morning:	
Stress Level yesterday and this morning:	

Day Seventeen: Test exercise up to 30 minutes

Start working on your menus for days 21-25

Plan Menu for Day	What you actually ate:
Breakfast • Flax granola with ½ portion fruit	
Lunch • Carrot Ginger Soup- optional • Salad with 15 grams of vegetarian protein	
Snack - Any Approved Snack	
Dinner • Approved protein • Sautéed kale with yellow squash, leeks • Any approved lettuce with herbs of choice	

Results	
Date:	
Supplements and medications on or recommended:	
Plan Day Followed yesterday:	
Any menu deviations yesterday:	
Water consumed (ounces) yesterday:	
Hours Slept yesterday:	
Exercise yesterday:	
Weight (pounds) today:	
BBT (F) today:	
Digestion yesterday and this morning:	
Mood yesterday and this morning:	
Stress Level yesterday and this morning:	

Day Eighteen: Test new fruit or new restaurant

Plan Menu for Day	What you actually ate:
Breakfast • New Cereal with chia seeds, sunflower seeds and approved fruit Or • Blueberry pear compote	
Lunch • Basil escarole soup • Salad with 15 grams of vegetarian protein	
Snack • 1 oz low sodium or no salt potato chips with ⅛ cup homemade guacamole Or • New approved fruit	
Dinner • Test restaurant if did not test fruit	

Results	
Date:	
Supplements and medications on or recommended:	
Plan Day Followed yesterday:	
Any menu deviations yesterday:	
Water consumed (ounces) yesterday:	
Hours Slept yesterday:	
Exercise yesterday:	
Weight (pounds) today:	
BBT (F) today:	
Digestion yesterday and this morning:	
Mood yesterday and this morning:	
Stress Level yesterday and this morning:	

Day Nineteen: Test Exercise up to 30 minutes

Start working on your menus for days 21-25
Repeat favorite day thus far with most weight loss

Plan Menu for Day	What you actually ate:
Breakfast *. Repeat favorite day thus far with most weight loss*	
Lunch	
Snack	
Dinner	
Results	
Date:	
Supplements and medications on or recommended:	
Plan Day Followed yesterday:	
Any menu deviations yesterday:	
Water consumed (ounces) yesterday:	
Hours Slept yesterday:	
Exercise yesterday:	
Weight (pounds) today:	
BBT (F) today:	
Digestion yesterday and this morning:	
Mood yesterday and this morning:	
Stress Level yesterday and this morning:	

Day Twenty: No Test

Start working on your menus for days 21-25
Repeat favorite day thus far with most weight loss

Plan Menu for Day	What you actually ate:
Breakfast *. Repeat favorite day thus far with most weight loss*	
Lunch	
Snack	
Dinner	

Results	
Date:	
Supplements and medications on or recommended:	
Plan Day Followed yesterday:	
Any menu deviations yesterday:	
Water consumed (ounces) yesterday:	
Hours Slept yesterday:	
Exercise yesterday:	
Weight (pounds) today:	
BBT (F) today:	
Digestion yesterday and this morning:	
Mood yesterday and this morning:	
Stress Level yesterday and this morning:	

Recipes

Breakfasts

Apple Streusel (V) (GF)

10 grams protein per serving Serves: 4

Streusel Topping

- 1½ cup almond flour
- 2 Tbsp brown sugar
- 1 tsp cinnamon
- ¼ cup avocado oil

Apple Filling

- 3 apples, cored and chopped into ½-inch pieces
- 1 Tbsp brown sugar
- 1 tsp cinnamon
- ½ tsp cardamom
- ¼ tsp cloves
- 4 eight oz. baking ramekins

Preheat oven to 350°F (175°C). In a small bowl mix all ingredients for streusel topping by hand or with hand mixer.

In a medium bowl combine all apple filling ingredients and mix well. Add apple mixture to mason jars and pack down with ½ inch of streusel topping.

Bake for 25-30 minutes until streusel topping is lightly browned. Serve warm or refrigerate. Top with almond slivers or 2 Tbsp chia.

Blueberry Pear Compote (V) (GF)

(Makes 2-3 servings)
- 1 cup blueberries
- 1 ripe pear
- 1-1¼ cups water (for extra yumminess you can use Silk coco milk instead! Can do ¾ cup water and ¾ cup coco milk)
- ½ cup chia seeds
- ⅛ cup almond slivers (omit if reactive to almonds)
- 1 Tbsp agave
- Cinnamon to taste- suggested ½ tsp can add cardamom, nutmeg, cloves too (all great digestives)

Chop the blueberries and pear and let simmer for 8-10 minutes in a pot of water (or coco milk) with cinnamon and agave.

Remove pot from heat and add chia seeds and stir frequently for 2 minutes. You can serve warm or refrigerate for later. The compote can also be frozen so feel free to make big batches!

Brunch Frittata "Muffins" (GF)

How much do I love this recipe? These egg muffins freeze very well, as do most of my breakfasts, saving you precious time.

Eggs are great for vegetarians as it's an excellent source of vitamin B12. This is so important for energy levels and thyroid health. B12 helps to produce red blood cells and offset anemia. It's also a vital nutrient to improve mood and fight depression.

Originally cow's milk was only from A2 cows, but most of what is commercially available in the United States is from A1 cows. The A2 protein is closer to the proteins in breast milk, goat and sheep milk, making it easier to digest for many. 8 large eggs

- ¼ cup whole milk (A2) or coconut milk
- ¼ cup broccoli florets
- 2 tsp finely chopped chives
- ½ tsp celery seed
- ½ tsp chipotle
- ½ tsp salt
- ½ tsp freshly ground black pepper
- ¾ cup grated Manchego
- ¼ cup chopped red onions
- Small basil leaves for garnish, optional

Preheat the oven to 350°F (175°C). Line a standard-sized, 12-well muffin pan with baking paper cups. Whisk the eggs and milk until well blended, then mix in the broccoli, chives, and spices. Place approximately 2 Tbsp of Manchego at the bottom of each muffin cup, and one teaspoon of the red onion, then evenly distribute the egg mixture among them so that each cup is about three-quarters full. Bake (middle rack) for about 30 minutes, until the frittatas are set. Serve immediately, garnish with basil, if desired. Alternatively, allow them to cool to room temperature before storing or freezing.

Carrot Chia Muffins (GF)

- 2¾ cups blanched almond flour
- ½ tsp baking soda
- 3 eggs
- ¼ cup chia seeds
- 6 Tbsp butter
- ⅛ cup raisins
- 1 tsp vanilla
- 1¼ cups finely grated or shredded carrot
- 1 Tbsp cinnamon
- ½ tsp ground ginger
- ¼ tsp ground cloves

Preheat oven to 350°F (175°C). Combine all the ingredients in a food processor and blend until thoroughly mixed, or for approximately 2 minutes. Pour the mixture into the paper-lined muffin cups and bake for approximately 22–25 minutes.

Cheddar Chive Muffin (GF)

Here is another option for your savory breakfast folks! It is gluten-free, low in sugar, and rich in protein. Goat cheese is much easier to digest than cow's cheese, as the molecules are smaller than cow's milk. Goat cheese is a better environmental option as well. Goats are smaller, take up less space, and eat less food. The foods they do eat are much more varied (weeds, herbs, shrubs, etc.), which is probably why goat milk is higher in nutrients.

- 4 cups blanched almond flour
- ½ tsp baking soda
- 4 large eggs
- 3 Tbsp chopped chives or scallions
- 2 cups grated goat cheddar cheese, Manchego, or goat gouda

Using a food processor, combine the almond flour and baking soda. Pulse in eggs until well combined. Briefly pulse in chives and cheddar cheese. Scoop a heaping ¼ cup of batter into each paper-lined muffin cup. Bake at 350°F (175°C) for 25–30 minutes. Serve warm or let cool and freeze.

Chia Fruit Jam (V) (GF)

Got fruit ready to go bad? This is the perfect rescue and a great way to take advantage of summer and fall bounty. This also makes great dessert topping.

Chia is incredibly rich in fiber. One ounce contains 10 grams, and the mucilage it releases greatly aids digestion. Foods that are high in fiber help people to feel full for longer, and a high fiber diet have been shown to help with weight loss. Increased fiber intake has been shown to lower blood pressure and cholesterol levels. Fiber also helps to regulate the immune system and lower inflammation

- 1 cup fruit
- 2 Tbsp chia seeds
- 2 Tbsp lemon juice or water
- 1 Tbsp agave

Add the fruit and chia in a bowl with lemon juice or water and agave. Let it sit for 30 minutes. You may add more fruit for more thickness. Serve on bread or a dessert topping. It's great with ice cream!

Flax Granola (V) (GF)

- 1 cup whole flax seeds
- ½ cup water
- cinnamon, nutmeg clove to taste
- Optional: pure vanilla extract raisins, walnuts, cranberries, etc. to taste (please be sure to include only nuts you have tested)

Soak 1 cup of flax overnight in the fridge in roughly ½ cup of water with cinnamon.

Spread in a thin layer on a baking sheet and bake at 275°F (135°C). Turn several times to dry out.

Optional add raisins and nuts of choice last 10 minutes. Should bake in 50-60 min.

Rice Pudding (V) (GF)

- 2 cups cooked basmati rice
- 1 cup coconut milk or rice milk
- ¼ cup raisins
- 1 tsp cinnamon
- ½ tsp cardamom
- ½ tsp nutmeg
- ½ tsp rose water or vanilla extract
- ½ cup crushed pecans or almond slivers

Using a medium-sized saucepan over low heat, combine all the ingredients and simmer, stirring frequently for 3 to 4 minutes, until well mixed and fragrant. Top with pecans and enjoy immediately.

The Plan Smoothie (V) (GF)

(Makes 1 serving)
- 1 ripe pear
- ½ cup berries
- ¼ avocado
- ¼ cup chia
- Rice Dream (RD) or Silk Coconut Milk (SCM)
- Optional: 1 tsp honey or agave
- Optional: vanilla extract or cinnamon

Fill Blender with enough RD or SCM to fill to 16 or 20 oz.

Blend. Ice is not recommended if you have thyroid dysfunction.

Vegan Breakfast Hash (V) (GF)

- 3 Medium Potatoes, chopped
- 1 Yellow Onion, chopped
- 2 carrots, grated
- 1 Zucchini, chopped
- ½ cup Shitake mushrooms, sliced
- ½ tsp Garlic Powder
- ½ tsp Cumin Powder
- ½ tsp Chipotle powder
- Salt and Pepper to Top
- 2-3 Tbsp Evoo

In a large pan over medium heat, add oil and diced potatoes. Stir potatoes and oil together and cook, covered, for about 10 minutes or until they begin to crisp and are softer when poked with a fork. Add the remaining ingredients and cook until tender, appx 5-6 minutes.

Warm Cranberry Flax Cereal (V) (GF)

Flax granola is a Plan favorite. It's amazing for digestion, thanks to its mucilage, and is also a great source of protein, calcium, and omega 3. But making the Flax granola is a bit time consuming, so this quick recipe is perfect for the time crunched. It's a hearty and warming breakfast. Please make to limit flax consumption to twice weekly as it's a phytoestrogen.

- 1 cup flaxseed
- 1 cup water
- ½ cup coconut milk or rice milk
- ¼ cup dried cranberries
- 1 Tbsp honey
- 1 tsp cinnamon
- ½ tsp cardamom
- ½ tsp ginger

Soak the flax in water overnight in a bowl. The next day, add 1 cup of soaked flax to coconut milk or rice milk, cranberries, honey, cinnamon, cardamom, and ginger in a saucepan. Simmer for 1-2 minutes. Serve warm.

Appetizers, Soups and Side Dishes

Arepas (Corn-Free) (GF)

- 1 cup blanched almond flour
- ½ cup water
- 2 eggs
- ½ cup grated Manchego
- 4 Tbsp EVOO (divided)

Toppings (optional):
- Guacamole, shiitake or maitake mushrooms, or grilled vegetables

Whisk all the ingredients together except EVOO and toppings and let sit for 5 minutes.

Heat a medium-sized skillet and add 1 tablespoon of EVOO.

Turn the heat to low and pour in ¼ of the batter.

Cook until browned on one side (3-4 minutes), repeating the process on the other side.

Repeat to make 4–6 arepas. Serve warm with optional toppings.

Asian Roasted Carrots and Broccoli (V) (GF)

- 3 Tbsp coconut aminos
- 1 Tbsp brown sugar, packed
- 1 Tbsp grated ginger
- 1 tsp rice vinegar
- 1 tsp Sriracha, or more, to taste
- 1 lb. carrots
- 1 Tbsp Evoo
- 3 cloves garlic, minced
- 1lb broccoli florets

Preheat oven to 375°F (190°C).

Lightly oil a baking sheet or coat with evoo.

In a small bowl, whisk together coconut aminos, brown sugar, ginger, garlic, rice vinegar and Sriracha; set aside.

Place carrots and broccoli in a single layer onto the prepared baking sheet. Drizzle with olive oil and sprinkle with garlic.

Place into oven and bake for 20-25 minutes, or until tender.

Stir in sauce mixture and gently toss to combine. Serve immediately, garnished with sesame seeds, if desired.

Basil Escarole Soup (V) (GF)

- 1 large white onion, fine diced
- ⅛ cup dried basil
- ½ tsp pink Himalayan Sea salt
- 1 tsp black pepper
- ¼ cup evoo
- 1-liter homemade stock or water
- 1 liter water
- 1 tsp agave or honey
- 2 lbs. carrots, chopped
- 8 cups zucchini pasta or 8 cups chopped zucchini, small
- 2 heads escarole, chopped

In a large soup pot sauté onion and basil in evoo. Add sea salt and black pepper and let simmer for 20 minutes. Add liquids, carrots and zucchini and let simmer for 20 minutes.

Add chopped escarole and let simmer an additional 10 minutes. Top with lemon or lime juice.

Braised Fennel (V) (GF)

- 1 large fennel bulb or 2 small bulbs
- 2 Tbsp butter
- 1 small clove garlic, whole
- ½ tsp thyme
- Sea salt and freshly ground black pepper
- ¼ cup dry white wine

Trim stalks flush with fennel bulb and cut each bulb lengthwise into quarters, or halves, if using small bulbs. In a heavy saucepan large enough to hold the fennel flat in one layer, melt 1 tablespoon butter over moderate heat. Add fennel, garlic, thyme, and toss to coat with butter. Season with salt and pepper, to taste. Add wine. Reduce heat to a simmer and cover. Braise for 10-15 minutes, or until vegetables are tender. Stir in remaining tablespoon butter and salt and pepper, to taste.

Butternut Squash Puree (V) (GF)

- 4 cups butternut squash, peeled, seeded and cut into 1-inch cubes (1 large)
- 1 cup homemade veggie broth
- 1 garlic clove
- ¼ cup coconut milk
- ¼ tsp sea salt
- ¼ tsp dried thyme

In medium saucepan, combine squash, broth and garlic and turn to medium-high heat. Bring to a boil and cover. Cook until squash is very tender, 15 to 20 minutes.

Transfer contents of the saucepan (do not drain) to a blender or food processor. Add the coconut milk, salt and thyme and puree in 20-second increments, scraping down the sides after each blending session. Blend until very smooth. Return puree to the saucepan and cover to keep warm until ready to serve

Carrot Ginger Soup (V) (GF)

- 1 Tbsp cinnamon
- 1 Tbsp cumin
- 1 Tbsp freshly ground black pepper
- 1 tsp ground cloves
- 1 tsp cardamom
- ½ tsp turmeric
- ½ tsp allspice
- 7 quarts water
- 2 Tbsp extra-virgin olive oil
- 5 lbs. carrots, chopped
- 2 large red onions, chopped
- 3 large zucchini, chopped
- 8 cloves of garlic, peeled
- 5–6 inches of ginger, peeled

Add the cinnamon, cumin, black pepper, cloves, cardamom, turmeric, and allspice to a dry skillet and sauté, stirring constantly for 30 seconds. Add 7 quarts water to large soup pot. Add the carrots, onion, zucchini, garlic, and ginger to the water and then add toasted spices. Bring the water to a boil and then let simmer for 45 minutes until the carrots are soft. Reserve 2 quarts of water for future soup stocks. Blend the carrot soup in batches.

Yield: 5 quarts, about 10–16 servings
Note: *Add 1 can of full-fat coconut milk and 5–6 Vietnamese chili peppers for a creamier, spicier soup!*

Carrot Zucchini Fritters

- 1 cup all-purpose flour, more as needed
- 2 tsp baking soda
- 1 tsp coriander
- ¾ tsp sea salt, more for serving
- 1 cup coconut or rice milk, more as needed
- 1 large egg
- ¼ tsp grated organic lemon zest
- ¼ tsp pepper
- 2 large carrots, grated (about 1½ cups)
- 1 large zucchini, grated (about 2 cups)
- 2 scallions, finely chopped
- 1 garlic clove, finely chopped
- ½ cup homemade coconut milk yogurt (page 83) OR ⅓ cup chevre and 3 Tbsp water mixed
- 1 Tbsp chopped mint
- 1 Tbsp extra-virgin olive oil
- Olive oil, for frying

In a large bowl, whisk together the flour, baking soda, coriander and ½ teaspoon salt. Whisk Then add together the milk, egg, lemon zest and pepper.
Add carrots, zucchini, and scallions. Allow to rest for 30 minutes.

To make the yogurt dip: in a food processor add the garlic, yogurt, mint and 1 tablespoon extra-virgin oil. Cover and refrigerate until ready to use.

Fill a wide saucepan with 1 inch of olive oil. Drop fritters by the tablespoon into the oil, being sure not to overcrowd the pan. Fry, turning occasionally, until golden all over, about 3 to 4 minutes. Use a slotted spoon to transfer fritters to the cookie sheet to drain. Transfer fritters to a platter or plate; serve.

Chicken Kale Soup (GF)

- 1 large white onion, chopped
- ⅛ cup dried basil
- ½ tsp pink Himalayan Sea salt
- 1 tsp black pepper
- ½ tsp dried sage
- 3 liters water
- 1 tsp agave or honey
- 2 lbs. carrots, chopped
- 8 cups packed kale chopped
- 2 chicken thighs with the bone
- ¼ cup lime juice to finish

Add all ingredients to a soup pot, bring to a boil and then let simmer for 45 minutes. Take out chicken. Portion soup into 16oz containers. Then remove chicken from bone and

shred. Add one ounce of shredded chicken to each 16 oz container of soup. This is low reactive and will not test like 2 animal proteins!

Coconut Yogurt (V) (GF)

- 1 can (15-16 oz) coconut milk
- 2 Capsules probiotics

Mix the two ingredients together in a glass jar and cover with cheese cloth. Let sit at room temperature for 2 days to ferment.

Refrigerate; keeps for five days. Enjoy!

Cream of Broccoli Soup (V) (GF)

- 3 Tbsp avocado oil
- 1 large onion chopped
- ½ tsp celery seed (dried)
- 2 cups homemade broth or water
- 2 cups water
- 1 can coconut milk
- 10 cups broccoli, chopped (about 5 heads of broccoli)
- 4 cups zucchini, chopped (about 2 medium zucchini)
- 1 Tbsp Sriracha -optional
- Ground black pepper to taste

Sautee onion and spices in 3 tablespoons of oil. Add in coconut milk, water and chicken broth along with the broccoli and zucchini and cook until vegetables are tender.

Serve immediately, or store and refrigerate up to 5 days.

Crockpot Pinto Beans- Chaat Masala (V) (GF)

- 2 cups pinto beans
- 4 cups water or homemade vegetable broth
- 1 Package Chaat Masala
- 8 cups chopped kale
- 2 cups chopped onions
- ½ inch piece of kombu (optional but helps to make beans more digestible)

Rinse dried pintos under cool water and drain

Put them into a large bowl and cover with hot water and let sit overnight.

In the morning, rinse beans well with cool water, drain and then put in crock pot.

Add chicken broth and all other ingredients.

Fill with water till water is about an inch or 2 above beans.

Cook on low all day for about 8-9 hours.

Remove kombu when done.

Endive Chowder (V) (GF)

- 6 endives
- 2 Tbsp evoo
- 2 leeks, chopped
- 2 shallots, diced
- ½ lb. yellow-fleshed potatoes, peeled and cut
- into small dice
- ½ lb. fennel chopped
- 2 large carrots, peeled and diced
- 2 tsp chopped fresh thyme
- 1 bay leaf
- 5 cups homemade broth or water
- 1 salt, plus more as needed
- 1 cup coconut milk
- Freshly ground white pepper, to taste
- 1 Tbsp finely chopped fresh chives
- 1 tsp finely chopped fresh tarragon

Reserve 8 outer leaves from the endives, then quarter and coarsely chop the remainder.

In a soup pot over medium-high heat, add evoo. Add the chopped endive, the leeks, shallots, potatoes, fennel, carrots, thyme, and bay leaf. Cook, stirring frequently, until the vegetables are fragrant, and the bottom of the pot is lightly glazed, about 7 minutes.

Add the broth. Bring to a boil, reduce the heat to low, cover and simmer until the potatoes are very soft, about 25 minutes. Remove the bay leaf. Mash a few of the vegetables against the side of the pot or transfer 1 to 2 cups to a blender and puree, then return to the pot. Add the cream and coconut milk, season with white pepper. Taste and season with salt, if needed. Stir in half the chives and tarragon. Finely sliver the reserved endive leaves and garnish the soup.

Hasselback Butternut Squash (V) (GF)

- 1 Small Butternut Squash
- 2 Tbsp Avocado oil
- 2 Garlic Cloves minced
- 2 Tbsp Honey or maple syrup
- 1 tsp onion powder
- 3-4 Sprigs Fresh thyme picked
- Sea salt and freshly ground pepper

Preheat oven to 400°F (205°C).

Start by cutting the butternut squash evenly in half on lengthwise. Scoop out the inside and discard. Place the halves on a baking sheet, cut side down.

In a small bowl whisk melted butter, with honey, garlic, onion powder, and thyme.

Brush the squash with half of the garlic butter mixture and sprinkle with salt and pepper.

Roast in the oven for 20-25 minutes. Remove from oven and allow to cool until ready to handle.

Place the squash halves to a cutting board and using a very sharp knife, slice it thinly, but not all the way through. Return the squash to the same baking sheet and brush with the remaining garlic butter mixture.

Return to the oven for and roast for an additional 15-20 minutes. or until golden brown on the tops and tender.

Hasselback Potatoes with Kale and Pesto (V) (GF)

- Hasselback potatoes
- 4 lbs. red potatoes or
- ⅓ cup olive oil
- Sea salt
- black pepper
- 1 bunch fresh thyme, leaves picked
- 6 cups kale deveined and chopped
- 1 small red onion chopped in rounds
- ½ cup sunflower pesto

Preheat the oven to 400°F (205°C). Wash and scrub the potatoes. Slice each potato thinly. Let each slice cut about two-thirds into the potato, leaving the bottom intact. Arrange in a circle. Sprinkle thyme over the potatoes. Drizzle olive oil, sea salt and pepper over potatoes. Bake for 30 minutes and then brush the potatoes with the remaining olive oil.

Add small amounts of kale and onions in between the layers of potato. Bake another 30 minutes. Drizzle pesto over the potatoes and kale and serve immediately, while still hot.

Herbed Cheese Wafers (GF)

- ¾ cup butter, softened
- ½ cup grated parmesan
- ⅓ cup crumbled chevre
- 1 Tbsp minced fresh tarragon or 1 tsp dried tarragon
- ½ tsp dried oregano
- 1 small garlic clove, minced
- 2 cups all-purpose flour

In a large bowl, beat butter, cheeses, tarragon, oregano and garlic until well mixed. Beat in flour (the dough will be crumbly).

Shape into a 14-in. roll. Wrap tightly and refrigerate for 4 hours or overnight.

Cut into ¼-in. slices; place on ungreased baking sheets.

Bake at 375°F (190°C) until golden brown and crisp, 10-12 minutes. Cool on wire racks.

Herby Pea Salad (V) (GF

- 1 Tbsp Evoo
- 2 medium leeks thinly sliced
- 3 small zucchini, halved and sliced
- 1 fennel, cut into pieces
- 3 cups frozen petite peas (about 16 ounces), thawed
- 2 Tbsp each minced fresh chives and parsley
- 1 to 2 Tbsp minced fresh tarragon

Dressing:

- 3 Tbsp Evoo
- 2 Tbsp balsamic
- 1 Tbsp fresh basil chopped
- 1 Tbsp fresh mint chopped
- 1 garlic clove minced
- ¼ tsp pepper

In a large skillet, heat oil over medium heat. Add leeks and fennel; cook and stir 4-6 minutes or until tender. Add peas and zucchini cooking for 5-6 minutes. Remove and immediately drop into ice water. Drain and pat dry and place in medium bowl. Whisk dressing ingredients. Pour over salad; toss to coat. Serve immediately.

Lemongrass Coconut Curry Soup with 'Zoodles' (V) (GF)

- 1 Tbsp avocado oil
- 1 stalk lemongrass, diced
- 1 Tbsp Thai green curry paste (page 138)
- 1 clove garlic, finely chopped
- ½ tsp minced fresh ginger
- ⅛ tsp cayenne
- 2 cups vegetable broth
- 1 cup onions
- ½ cup water
- 2 medium zucchini, cut with a spiralizer (zoodles)
- 1 cup sliced shitake mushrooms
- 1 cup carrots, chopped
- ⅓ cup scallions, diced
- 1 tsp sea salt
- ½ tsp ground black pepper
- ½ cup basil chopped
- 2 Tbsp lime juice

Heat a saucepan over medium heat. Add oil, lemongrass, green curry paste, garlic, ginger, onion and cayenne. Cook until fragrant, about 3 minutes. Add broth and water to the saucepan with the lemongrass mixture and bring to a boil. Add vegetables and simmer for 4-5 minutes until vegetables are tender. Season soup with salt and pepper. Add basil. Stir to combine, adjust seasoning if needed, and ladle into bowls.

Maaqouda

- 2 lb. potatoes
- 2 eggs, beaten
- ½ cup panko
- ½ tsp garlic powder
- ½ tsp onion powder
- 3 Tbsp finely chopped oregano
- ½ tsp turmeric
- ½ tsp cumin
- Flour (for coating)
- Sea salt
- Pepper
- Avocado oil for frying
- Lemon wedges

Bring a large pot of salted water to a boil and cook the potatoes with their skin for at least 30 minutes or until tender.

Mash potatoes and add the panko, garlic, onion, cumin, turmeric, oregano, beaten eggs, salt and pepper. Stir to incorporate all the ingredients. If the mixture is too firm, add more panko.

Shape 2-inch diameter patties.

In a large saucepan, add oil. Drench Maaqouda in flour to cover both sides.

Remove excess flour and deep fry on one side, then the other. Drain on paper towels and serve with lemon.

Oregano and Cheese Bread

Oregano is one of my favorite herbs. First, it grows like a weed, so I look like some magical gardener. Second, it has such incredible health benefits, from boosting your immune system to being antifungal and anti-inflammatory. It's also a yeast fighter. This recipe is for a bread maker (I am so in love with mine), but you could easily alter this recipe so that you won't have to use one.

- 3 cups bread flour
- 1 cup water
- ½ cup freshly grated cheese (Romano or Parmesan)
- 3 Tbsp sugar
- 1 Tbsp dried-leaf oregano
- 1½ Tbsp EVOO
- 1 tsp salt
- 2 tsp active dry yeast

Prepare the bread in the bread machine using the dough cycle. Once finished, bake in a preheated 375°F (190°C) oven for 25 to 30 minutes or until golden brown.

Parmesan-Roasted Broccoli (GF)

- 8 cups broccoli florets
- 4 garlic cloves, peeled and thinly sliced
- Evoo
- 1 tsp Sea salt
- ½ tsp freshly ground black pepper
- 2 tsp organic grated lemon zest
- 2 Tbsp freshly squeezed lemon juice
- 3 Tbsp sun seeds toasted
- ⅓ cup freshly grated Parmesan cheese
- 2 Tbsp julienned fresh basil leaves

Preheat the oven to 375°F (190°C).

Place the broccoli florets on a sheet pan large enough to hold them in a single layer.

Toss the garlic on the broccoli and drizzle with 5 tablespoons olive oil.

Sprinkle with the salt and pepper.

Roast for 20 to 25 minutes, until crisp-tender and the tips of some of the florets are browned.

Remove the broccoli from the oven and immediately toss with 1 ½ tablespoons olive oil, the lemon zest, lemon juice, sun seeds, Parmesan, and basil. Serve hot.

Parmesan Kale Chips (GF)

- 1 bunch kale
- 2 Tbsp olive oil
- Sea Salt
- 2 Tbsp grated Parmesan cheese

Preheat oven to 177°C (350°F (175°C)). Wash and dry the kale. Cut leaves from the ribs (discard ribs).

In a large bowl toss kale with olive oil and salt to taste.

Place kale on a cookie sheet, ensuring that the leaves are well-spaced to prevent them from steaming instead of crisping. Bake until crispy, checking periodically, 10 to 20 minutes.

Remove from oven and sprinkle with cheese.

Plan Trail Mix (V) (GF)

- ⅛ cup raw sunflower seeds
- 1 Tbsp dried cranberries

Combine. Enjoy.

Potato Kugel (GF)

- ½ cup EVOO
- 3 eggs
- 1 TSP Himalayan Sea Salt
- ½ tsp freshly ground black pepper
- 6 large Red Potatoes or Yukon Gold Potatoes
- 1 large onion, quartered.
- 1 TBL Chopped fresh chives

Preheat oven to 425°F (220°C). Place either your cupcake tins, 4oz to 6oz ramekins on a baking sheet and place in preheated oven on middle rack to heat while preparing everything. This step is important, so the outside gets crispy.

Fill a large bowl with cold water and as you peel the potatoes, place them in cold water to prevent them from browning.

Beat the eggs in a small bowl and add salt and pepper. Mix well until frothy, about 1 minutes.

In a small saucepan over medium-low heat, pour ¾ cup EVOO in and warm.

Shred the potatoes in a food processor fitted with a shredding disk. Removing the potatoes as your work cutting them in half to fit the food processor chute. Return the shredded potatoes to the cool water and let stand for 5 to 6 minutes. Drain them and place on a clean kitchen towel squeezing out as much liquid as possible. Transfer to a large bowl.

In the same food processor bowl, shred the onions. Drain them in a fine-mesh strainer gently pressing to remove the excess liquid and add them to the bowl with the potatoes.

Add the egg mixture and the heated oil from the stove top and mix very well. Add ½ TBL of the chives.

Carefully remove the heated cups from the oven and oil using a pastry brush use the remaining ¼ cup of EVOO and spread evenly over the bottom and sides of your dish until well covered.

Spoon the potato mixture evenly into the hot, oiled cups smoothing the top with the back of a spoon.

If using glass or ceramic ramekins, bake for 1 hour. If the sides are still pale, cook an additional 20 minutes until the tops look crunchy and the sides look golden and brown. IF USING CUPCAKE TIN, check after 45 minutes as metal will brown faster. If not brown and crunchy, cook an additional 10 minutes and keep checking until done.

Loosen the edges with a knife and unmold. Sprinkle with remaining chives and serve.

Roasted Fennel with Manchego and Wild Rice (GF)

- 3 to 4 fennel bulbs (reserve fronds for garnish and soup stock), chopped
- 2 large yellow squash, chopped
- 2 cups butternut squash, chopped in cubes.
- 1 large red onion, chopped
- About 1 cup EVOO
- Fresh ground black pepper
- 1 tsp sage
- 1 cup grated Manchego
- 4 cups cooked wild rice, cooked with ½ cup dried cranberries
- Pecans for topping

Preheat the oven to 375°F (190°C).

Trim off the tough outer layer of each fennel bulb. Cut each bulb in half from top to bottom, then cut each half into 2 equal wedges, keeping the core intact; this will help hold the wedges together.

Pour enough oil to generously cover the bottom of the baking sheet, then add the fennel wedges, onion, yellow squash and butternut squash.

Sprinkle each wedge with pepper and sage. Top each one with the cheese. Bake for about 30 minutes or until the fennel is tender enough to be easily pierced with a fork and the cheese is golden brown.

Garnish with the fronds and serve warm with wild rice, top with pecans

Sautéed Fennel and Snow Peas with Shitake (V) (GF)

- 1 lb. Fennel
- 1 lb. Snow peas
- 3 Tbsp Evoo
- Sea salt
- Ground black pepper
- ½ lb. shitakes
- 2 Tbsp pumpkin seeds
- 4 cups basmati rice

Preheat the oven to 375°F (190°C).

Cut the stalks and fronds off the fennel. Then cut the fennel bulb into small wedges. Arrange in a baking dish. Drizzle olive oil on top. Salt and pepper to taste.

Bake in the oven for 30 minutes or until the fennel has turned a nice golden color.

While the fennel is baking, Add the snow peas and shitakes to a medium skillet over medium heat. Cook for 3-4minutes until tender. Remove from pan and add the pumpkin seeds. Toast for one minute. Remove the fennel and add to the snow peas. Serve over rice.

Smashed Cucumber and Carrot Salad (V) (GF)

- 1-pound seedless cucumbers (Japanese or Persian the best but English will work as well) rinsed and dried
- ½ tsp sea salt
- 2 medium carrots, peeled into noodles with a vegetable peeler
- ¼ cup stir fry sauce (recipe below)
- 1 garlic clove, minced
- ½ tsp sesame oil (test)
- ¼ tsp crushed red chili pepper TEST or ⅛ tsp red pepper
- 2 green onions, thinly sliced
- 2 tsp toasted sesame seeds TEST can omit

Place the cucumbers on a large cutting board and gently smash them with a meat pounder, cleaver, or small cast iron skillet until they split open.

Trim the ends and cut the bashed cucumbers into bite-size pieces. Grab a fine-mesh strainer or a colander that fits in a medium bowl.

Transfer the cucumber pieces to the colander and toss with the salt.

Place the strainer and bowl with the salted cucumbers in the fridge while you prepare the other ingredients. (You can salt the for as short as 5 minutes and as long as 4 hours).

Whisk together the stir-fry sauce, minced garlic, sesame oil and crushed red chili pepper.

Grab the drained cucumbers out of the fridge and put them in a bowl with the carrot noodles and most of the green onions. Add the dressing and toss well. Top with sesame seeds if using and the rest of the green onions.

Snow Pea Salad (V) (GF)

- Earl Grey Tea Vinaigrette:
- 2 earl grey tea bags
- ¼ cup boiling water
- ½ tsp agave syrup
- 1 tsp grated fresh ginger
- Salad:
- 4 cups arugula
- 2 medium carrots, grated
- 2 cups snow peas steamed and chilled.
- ¼ cup almond slivers

Vinaigrette:

Steep tea bags in hot water in a small dish for about 1 hour. Squeeze tea out of tea bags. Whisk in dressing ingredients.

Salad:

Toss together greens, shredded carrots, and snow peas in a large salad bowl. Toss in vinaigrette. Sprinkle with almond slivers. Serve immediately.

Spinach Soufflé (GF)

- Oil for casserole dish
- 2 tsp EVOO (for frying)
- 6 cups packed spinach
- ⅓ cup thinly sliced scallions
- 1½ cups manchego (grated)
- 8 eggs (beaten)
- 2 Tbsp chopped fresh dill
- 1 tsp tarragon
- 1 tsp black pepper

Preheat the oven to 375°F (190°C). Oil an 8½-inch by 12-inch casserole dish.

Heat the oil in a large frying pan, add the spinach and scallions, and sauté until the spinach is wilted (about 2 minutes). Transfer the spinach to the casserole dish, and layer it with the grated cheese.

Beat the eggs together with cheese, dill and tarragon and pepper and pour the egg mixture over the spinach & scallion mixture.

Bake for about 35 minutes or until the mixture is completely set and is lightly browned. Let cool for about 5 minutes before serving.

Summer Squash with Turmeric Ghee (GF)

- 1-pound yellow summer squash, sliced on the bias into 1-inch thick slices
- Evoo for drizzling
- Sea salt
- 2 Tbsp ghee
- ½ tsp turmeric
- 1 tsp coriander
- 1 tsp honey
- ¼ cup skinless hazelnuts, toasted and roughly chopped

Place a medium skillet over medium-high heat. Add the squash and let them char a little, tossing often.

Drizzle in a little olive oil just to coat, and sauté until nearly crisp-tender.

Season with sea salt. Transfer the squash to a large bowl before continuing.

In a small pan over medium heat, add ghee and add the turmeric. Stir until the butter has melted and the turmeric is evenly distributed. Cook 1 minute.

Stir in the coriander, honey, and hazelnuts until combined. Return the squash back to the skillet and toss to combine. Serve immediately.

Sweet and Spicy Roasted Moroccan Carrots (V) (GF)

- 1 ½ lbs. whole carrots
- 2 Tbsp Evoo
- 1 Tbsp brown sugar
- ½ tsp salt
- ½ tsp pepper
- 1 Tbsp pomegranate juice
- ½ tsp organic orange zest
- ½ tsp cayenne
- ¼ tsp cumin
- ⅛ tsp cinnamon
- ¼ cup chopped basil

Preheat oven to 375°F (190°C). Chop carrots.

Cut in half length wise, and quarter the thicker pieces so all are relatively the same thickness (no bigger than ½ inch thick).

In a small bowl mix oil, sugar, salt, and pepper. Toss this with the carrots and spread out in a single layer on a sheet pan.

Cover and place in the oven for 15 minutes. Uncover and continue roasting 20 minutes more, stirring once halfway through. Roast until tender.

Whisk the juice, cayenne, cumin, and cinnamon. Toss with dressing with the roasted carrots and garnish with fresh basil and orange zest.

Timbale (GF)

This is a great dish to keep adding vegetables in as you test them!
- 1 head of kale
- 1 large zucchini
- 1 red onion
- ½ large carrots
- 4 oz goat cheese
- 2 oz parmesan or manchego
- 6 shiitakes

Preheat oven to 400°F (205°C).

Use a mandolin or slice vegetables as thinly as you can. Create layers like a lasagna: zucchini, onions, goat cheese, carrots, shitakes, Swiss chard, carrots, zucchini and top with parmesan.

Cook for 30 minutes or until top layer of cheese is slightly golden.

Zucchini-Noush (V) (GF)

I love babaganoush, but like many of my clients, I am reactive to eggplant. Subbing zucchini was a natural idea with this summer's bounty and thus was born zucchini-noush!

- ¼ cup extra virgin olive oil
- 1 large white onion chopped fine (approx. 2 cups)
- ¼ cup cumin
- 1 tsp pink Himalayan Sea salt
- ⅛ cup water
- 5 large zucchini chopped (approx. 10 cups) oil for baking sheet
- optional: 1 cup sunflower tahini

Add oil to a large skillet on medium heat and add onion, cumin and sea salt. Stir until spices are thoroughly mixed and then mix in water. Lower heat to lowest setting and let simmer for 30 minutes stirring often.

Add zucchini to the onion and mix well. Take zucchini/onion mixture and spread on a well-oiled baking sheet. Bake at 325°F (165°C) for 40 minutes.

Remove from zucchini from the oven and add to a medium mixing bowl. Mix well. The zucchini will break down to a chunky texture. Optional, add 1 cup sunflower tahini and mix well.

Main Course

Baked Cod Recipe with Lemon and Garlic

- 1 ½ lb. Cod fillet pieces, 4-6 pieces
- 2 Tbsp chopped oregano
- 2 Tbsp chopped thyme
- Lemon Sauce
- 5 Tbsp fresh lemon juice
- 5 Tbsp Evoo
- 2 Tbsp Butter or
- 5 garlic cloves, minced

For Coating

- ⅓ cup all-purpose flour
- 1 tsp ground coriander
- ¾ tsp ground cumin
- ¾ tsp salt
- ½ tsp black pepper

Preheat oven to 400°F (205°C).

Mix together the lemon juice, olive oil, and melted butter in a shallow bowl. Set aside. In another shallow bowl, mix the all-purpose flour, spices, salt and pepper. Set next to the lemon sauce.

Pat the fish dry. Dip the fish in the lemon sauce then dip it in the flour mixture. Shake off excess flour. Reserve the lemon sauce for later.

In a skillet add oil and cook fish on one side for 4-5 minutes. Add garlic to the lemon sauce. Drizzle all over the fish fillets. Flip fish on other side. Bake in the heated oven until fish is cooked approximately 6-8 minutes.

Charleston Chicken

- 1 (2 to 3-pound) whole chicken
- 1 tsp dried oregano
- 1 tsp garlic powder
- 1 Tbsp onion powder
- 1 tsp chipotle
- 1 tsp ground ginger
- 1 tsp dried sage
- 1 tsp sea salt
- 1 Tbsp freshly ground black pepper
- 2 cloves garlic, smashed
- 1 (12-ounce) can beer
- ½ pound bacon

Mix dry ingredients in small bowl. Rub half of the ingredients on inside cavity of chicken. Gently peel skin away from chicken and rub mixture into meat of chicken.

Open beer can pour out about ½ cup. Drop the garlic cloves into the beer can. Place chicken, open end down, over the beer can to insert the beer into the cavity.

Place chicken, standing up, in large sauté pan. Place one third of the bacon in the top cavity of the chicken and drape the remaining bacon down the outside of the chicken. Pierce the bacon to the chicken with toothpicks.

Place chicken in the oven for 10 minutes and then lower temperature to 325°F (165°C) and cook for another 1 hour, or until the internal temperature in the thickest part of the thigh reaches 165 degrees F on an instant-read thermometer.

Chinese Chicken and Broccoli (GF)

- 8 cups broccoli florets
- 4 cups yellow squash, chopped into cubes.
- 3 Tbsp Avo oil
- 6 boneless chicken thighs skinless
- 3 cloves garlic peeled and finely chopped
- 4 scallions, chopped
- 3 Tbsp grated ginger
- ½ cup coconut aminos
- ½ cup Chinese cooking wine

Heat a wok over a high heat and add a bit of oil.

Add the chicken and brown on all sides to seal the meat.

Remove the chicken and set aside.

Fry the garlic, spring onion and ginger for 30 seconds in the hot wok, adding a little more oil if necessary, tossing now and then.

Put the chicken back in the wok. Add the coconut aminos and cooking wine, squash, and broccoli. Cook for ten minutes or until chicken is done.

Cod with fennel and potato (GF)

- 3 cups potatoes, red potatoes, Yukon gold and fingerlings are least reactive
- 1.4 cup EVOO
- ½ cup thinly sliced fennel bulb (reserve some fronds for garnish)
- ½ cup thinly sliced scallions
- 2 TBL minced garlic
- 1 TBL chopped fresh tarragon
- 1 tsp chopped dill
- Himalayan Sea Salt
- ½ tsp freshly ground black pepper
- ½ cup dry white wine
- ½ cup homemade veg stock or water
- Six-6oz cod fillets (or any white fish)
- Lemon wedges (organic if possible)

Place potatoes in a small saucepan; cover with cold water by 1 inch. Bring to a simmer over medium-high heat and cook for 1 minute or until potatoes are not quite fully tender. Drain well; sprinkle with ¼ tsp salt and set aside.

Heat oil in a large skillet over medium-high heat. Add fennel, onion, garlic, tarragon, dill, ½ tsp salt and ¼ tsp pepper. Sauté 4 minutes or until the vegetables are tender. Add wine, stock, and lemon slices. Bring to a simmer. Sprinkle cod with ¼ tsp salt and ¼ tsp pepper. Add potatoes and cod to pan, nestling the cod into the sauce. Cover and reduce heat. Simmer 5 minutes or until fish is done.

Divide potato mixture evenly among 6 bowls (approx. ½ cup portion) Top each serving with 1 fish fillet and serve with lemon wedges.

Garnish with some reserved fennel fronds

Curry-spiced Potato Burgers (V)

- 2 medium russet potatoes (chopped)
- 5 Tbsp avocado oil
- 1½ cup finely diced broccoli
- ¾ cup finely diced fennel
- ¼ cup finely diced carrot
- ¼ cup Alco eats Creamy Spuds (or curry powder)
- 2 Tbsp coconut milk
- 1 tsp lime juice
- 1 cup breadcrumbs or panko (plus more for dredging)

Cook the potatoes in simmering water for 20 minutes.

Rinse to remove starch, then pat dry. Cool and then mash potatoes.

Pour 1 Tbsp of oil in a sauté pan on medium heat Add the diced vegetables and spices and sauté for 10–15 minutes.

Once the vegetables cool, add them to the potato mash. Add the lime juice to the potato mix.

Combine the panko with the potato and vegetable mixture and mix well.

Make 8 patties, roughly 3 inches round. Let sit for 10 minutes, then dredge patties in more panko.

Heat a skillet with 2 Tbsp of oil, placing 4 patties on it. Sauté the patties until browned and crunchy.

Serve immediately or freeze.

Duck Breast with Caramelized Nectarines (GF)

Duck breast:

- 1 duck breast
- Sea salt
- Pepper
- 1 Tbsp olive oil
- 1 garlic clove, halved
- 1 fresh rosemary sprig

Caramelized nectarines:

- 1 tsp Evoo
- 3 nectarines, cut into wedges
- 2 Tbsp honey
- ½ tsp cinnamon

Duck breast:

Place the duck breast on your work surface. Rub it with salt and pepper.

Heat the olive oil in an ovenproof skillet over medium heat. Add the garlic and rosemary in the process, to flavor the oil.

Turn the heat to medium-high, add the duck breast and fry it for 2 minutes on each side.

Transfer to the oven and bake for 8 minutes at 360ºF/180ºC.

Caramelized nectarines:

In a skillet over low heat add olive oil, honey, cinnamon, and the nectarines.

Cook and stir them shortly until tender.

Serve the duck breast sliced together with caramelized nectarine wedges. Drizzle everything with the drippings from the caramelization process.

Egg Roll Bowl (GF)

- 1 TBL avocado oil or EVOO
- 2 medium carrots, chopped
- 4 oz shiitake mushrooms stemmed and thinly sliced
- 4 garlic cloves minced
- 2 Tbsp finely minced red onion
- 1 TBL fresh ginger finely grated
- 2 pounds fresh ground chicken
- 1 small Napa cabbage cut in half and thinly sliced crosswise (Test)
- 2 TBL Coconut aminos
- 2 tsp rice vinegar
- 2 tsp sesame oil (REMEMBER THIS IS A TEST)
- Himalayan Sea Salt
- Siracha Optional to taste (start with 1 TBL)
- Fresh mint for garnish
- Scallions for garnish
- Black sesame seeds

In a 12" or larger skillet heat over medium heat and add oil. Once hot, toss in carrots, red onion and mushrooms. Sprinkle lightly with salt and sauté for 3 to 5 minutes.

Toss in garlic and ginger and stir fry for 30 seconds or until fragrant.

Add chicken and sauté until done

Transfer chicken with slotted spoon to another platter leaving the cooking liquid in the pan.

Throw cabbage into pan and sauté for 3 to 5 minutes until wilted

Lower heat to medium and add chicken back into skillet and stir to combine.

Season with the coconut aminos, rice vinegar and Sriracha if using. Taste and adjust with more seasoning if needed.

Sprinkle with scallions, sesame seeds and fresh mint and enjoy

Garlic Roast Whole Chicken (GF)

- 1 whole head garlic
- 1 chicken
- 1 bunch green onions, trimmed
- 1 cup coconut aminos
- 2 Tbsp grated ginger

Preheat the oven to 425°F (220°C)

Wipe the chicken. And then stuff the green onions into the chicken's cavity. Separate the skin over the breast and thighs from the meat. Slide the peeled garlic evenly under the skin. Add the ginger to the coconut aminos.

Set the bird into the roasting pan and put it in the oven. Roast for 15 minutes, then turn down the heat to 375°F (190°C). After 30 minutes, brush some of the paste or sauce over the chicken, being sure to coat the breast area thoroughly. Then continue roasting, basting the chicken every 15 minutes or so with the paste or sauce and then the juices.

Ginger Beef Stir Fry Recipe with Carrot Zoodles (GF)

Marinade:

- 2 Tbsp unseasoned rice vinegar
- ½ cup coconut aminos
- 2 Tbsp peeled, grated fresh ginger
- 1 tsp ground cumin
- ½ tsp cayenne

Beef and stir-fry:

- 1¼ to 1½ lbs. top sirloin steak, sliced in ½ inch thick strips
- 2 Tbsp avocado oil
- 4 scallions chopped
- 2 cloves garlic, thinly sliced
- 2-3 hot chilies, preferably red serranoes, seeded, sliced
- 3 Tbsp grated ginger
- ¼ cup chopped basil
- Carrot noodles- 10 cups

Marinate the beef:

In a medium bowl, whisk together the marinade ingredients; the coconut aminos, vinegar, grated ginger, cumin, and cayenne. Mix the beef in with the marinade to coat and let it sit for at least 30 minutes, and up to 4 hours, in the fridge.

Brown the beef strips:

Heat the oil in a wok or a large sauté pan, over high heat. As the oil is heating up, pat the beef dry and separate it into small batches. Working in batches, sauté beef until just brown outside but rare inside, no more than 1 minute. Transfer beef to a bowl.

Stir fry chilies, garlic, ginger: When all the beef is cooked, put the chilies and garlic into the pan and stir-fry 30-45 seconds. Add the julienned ginger and cook for 30-45 seconds more. Add the beef back to the pan. Add the scallions and carrot zoodles and mix everything together. Cook for 1-2 minutes. Remove from heat, add in basil. Serve beef over scallion carrots.

Honey Balsamic Lamb Chops (GF)

- • ⅓ cup balsamic vinegar
- • 1 garlic clove
- • 2 Tbsp honey
- • ⅓ cup avocado oil
- • ½ tsp Sea salt and fresh ground black pepper
- • 8 small lamb chops
- • 2 Tbsp EVOO
- • ½ Tbsp chopped fresh rosemary leaves

Pace a grill pan over medium-high heat or preheat a grill

In the bowl of a food processor, combine the balsamic vinegar, garlic and honey. Pulse until well blended. With the machine running, slowly pour in the oil until the mixture is smooth and forms a thick sauce.

Season the chops with the salt and pepper. Drizzle the chops with the olive oil and sprinkle with the rosemary. Grill the chops for 2 to 3 minutes per side until medium-rare.

Arrange the chops on a platter and spoon the sauce over the top or serve on the side.

Indonesian Tempeh with Kale & Gado Gado Sauce (V)

- Two 8 oz. tempeh
- 4 Tbsp EVOO
- 4 cups kale (deveined and chopped)
- 2 carrot (chopped)
- 1 yellow squash (chopped)
- 4 cups kale (deveined and chopped)
- ½ cup gado gado sauce (page 132)
- ½ papaya (chopped)

Marinade:
- 2 cloves crushed garlic
- 1 cup water
- ¼ cup coconut aminos
- 1 Tbsp fresh ginger (grated)
- 1 tsp cumin
- ½ tsp chipotle

Add the marinade ingredients to a bowl and mix well.

Slice the tempeh, 1-inch thick, and score both sides of the tempeh. Marinate the tempeh in the sauce for 20 minutes.

Remove tempeh from bowl and blot dry. Pan fry the tempeh in a skillet with oil, browning them on both sides. Remove from heat.

Add the chopped carrots and yellow squash to the skillet and sauté for 4-5 minutes. Then add kale to the skillet and sauté for another 2 minutes until wilted.

Place the vegetables on a platter and top with tempeh. Top with the gado gado sauce, then papaya.

Jamaican Jerk Chicken – Instapot (GF)

- 4 Pounds bone-in skin on chicken pieces (I like chicken thighs)
- 5 cloves garlic
- ⅓ cup fresh lime juice
- ½ cup coconut aminos
- 2 habanero peppers (omit for mild chicken) ** see notes for options
- 1 ½ inch piece of peeled fresh ginger
- 4 stalks green onion
- 1 tsp allspice
- ½ tsp ground cinnamon
- ¼ tsp ground nutmeg
- 3 green onions-sliced for garnish

Add the sauce ingredients (all except the chicken) to a blender and blend until combined.

Plug in your Instant Pot and press sauté button. Add 2 to 3 Tablespoons of avocado and allow to heat.

Place chicken on the hot surface, skin-side down and brown for 4 to 5 minutes or until chicken has a nice golden crisp on it. Flip the chicken to the other side and brown for another 2 minutes. (don't cook chicken through). You will need to do this in batches. Transfer browned chicken to a plate while you brown the rest.

Transfer all the chicken back into the pressure cooker and pour in the sauce. Press the "manual" button or Pressure Cook and set the time for 20 minutes. Make sure it is set to cook on high heat and that the relief valve is set to the sealed position.

When done, allow it to naturally release for at least one hour and up to 2 hours.

Open the lid and either serve immediately or transfer to the oven and broil to make the skin crispy.

Lamb Braised in Pomegranate (GF)

- 3 pounds lamb shoulder blade chops
- Sea salt and freshly ground pepper to taste
- 1 Tbsp avocado oil
- 1 onion, sliced
- 1 pinch salt
- 4 cloves garlic, sliced
- 2 cups pomegranate juice
- ⅓ cup balsamic vinegar
- ¼ tsp dried rosemary
- ¼ cup mint diced
- ¼ tsp cayenne
- 1 Tbsp honey, or more to taste
- 2 Tbsp pomegranate seeds
- 1 Tbsp fresh thyme chopped

Preheat oven to 300°F (150°C). Season lamb chops with salt and black pepper. Heat oil in a cast iron skillet over medium heat. Place lamb chops in skillet and cook until browned on all sides, about 8 minutes. Transfer lamb to a plate and reduce heat to medium. Stir onion and a pinch of salt into the skillet; cook until onions are slightly golden, about 3 minutes. Stir in garlic and cook for 30 seconds. Pour pomegranate juice in and scrape any browned bits off the bottom of the pot.

Pour in balsamic vinegar, increase heat to high, and bring to a boil. Stir rosemary, oregano, and cayenne into pomegranate juice mixture.

Reduce heat to medium and cook until the jus is reduced by half, about 10 minutes. Return lamb and any accumulated juices to skillet and spoon pomegranate mixture over lamb, and cover. Cook for 10 more minutes. Stir in honey and season with salt and black pepper to taste. Garnish with pomegranate seeds and thyme.

Lemon Grilled Scallop Skewers (GF)

- • ¼ cup of EVOO
- • 2 garlic cloves minced
- • 2 Tbsp lemon juice
- • ½ tsp sea salt
- • ½ tsp black pepper
- • 2-3 pounds sea scallops—ALWAYS DRY SCALLOPS
- •Extra lemon to grill along scallops

Make marinade: mix olive oil, garlic, lemon juice, salt and pepper in a bowl then toss in the scallops. (Add in any additions listed below)

Preheat grill or grill pan to medium-high heat

Cut the extra lemon

Remove the scallops from the marinade and slide 4 to 5 onto each skewer.

Cook the scallops for 2 to 3 minutes per side or until opaque

Rub a little oil on the cut halves of lemon and grill the alongside the scallops

Before serving squeeze that yummy smoky lemon juice over the scallops

Lentil Zucchini Fritters (V) (GF)

- 1 cup red lentils
- 1 medium to large zucchini
- ½ medium onion, thinly sliced
- ½ tsp sea salt
- ¼ tsp cayenne pepper
- ¼ tsp ground turmeric
- 1 cup basil
- 1 TBS lemon zest
- 1 cup avocado oil

Rinse lentils, then soak in 2 cups water at room temperature for at least 1 hour and up to 12. Soaking the lentils for this long will make them super-plump and tender which in turn makes them a lot easier to blend.

Meanwhile, trim ends of zucchini and cut crosswise into 3" pieces about 2" long. Cut each piece lengthwise into ¼"-thick planks. Stack a few planks and slice lengthwise into ¼"-thick matchsticks. Transfer zucchini to a colander set in a medium bowl. Add onion and salt to colander and toss to combine. Let zucchini and onion sit until about 1 TBS of liquid has released and the vegetables looked wilted and soft, 30 minutes to 2 hours (to maximize your downtime, do this while the lentils are soaking). Gently pat dry with paper towels to remove any excess moisture. The less moisture in the veggies, the less soggy your fritters will be, so be sure not to skip this step.

Drain lentils and transfer to a food processor. Add the red pepper, turmeric and ⅛ tsp salt. Pulse, scraping down sides until a puree forms. Transfer to a medium bowl and add zucchini and onion mixture, parsley or basil and lemon zest. Toss well with a rubber spatula to combine (it will look like too many vegetables for the lentils, but that's just what you want)

Heat avocado oil in a large cast-iron skillet over medium-high until a small amount of batter added to the fat sizzles. Carefully drop ¼ cup batter and flatten to a pancake with the back of a large metal spoon dipped into the hot oil to prevent sticking. Repeat 3 times for a total of 4 fritters. Fry until deep golden brown on one side, about 3 minutes. Turn with a slotted spatula and continue to fry until deep golden brown on the second side, about 3 minutes more. Transfer fritters to a wire rack set in a paper towel-lined baking sheet to drain. Season with salt if needed and repeat with remaining batter. You should have 8 to 10 fritters.

Optional: Serve with Plan Lemon Goat Cheese Dipping Sauce (page 133)

Pear and Pomegranate Lamb Tagine (GF)

- 2½ pounds lamb shanks
- 2 large pears, finely chopped
- 3 cups thinly sliced shallots
- 1 cup pomegranate juice, divided
- 1 Tbsp honey
- 1½ tsp ground cinnamon
- 1 tsp salt
- 1 tsp ground allspice
- 1 tsp ground cardamom
- ¼ cup pomegranate seeds
- ¼ cup minced herbs of choice

Place lamb in a 5- or 6-qt. oval slow cooker. Add pears and shallots.

Combine ½ cup pomegranate juice, honey, and seasonings; add to slow cooker.

Cook, covered, on low for until meat is tender, 6-8 hours.

Remove lamb to a rimmed serving platter; keep warm.

Stir remaining pomegranate juice into cooking liquid; pour over lamb.

Sprinkle with pomegranate seeds and herbs.

Psari Plaki Fish

- ½ cup olive oil
- 2 large onions (thinly sliced)
- 2 to 3 garlic cloves (minced)
- 1 tsp celery seed
- 5 plum tomatoes (seeded and diced)
- 3 pounds firm white fish fillets (such as cod, halibut, or flounder)
- Dash salt
- Dash fresh ground black pepper
- 2 tsp dried oregano
- 1 tsp thyme
- 2 organic lemons (thinly sliced)
- 3 Tbsp lemon juice
- ½ cup dry white wine
- ¼ cup panko

Preheat the oven to 350°F (175°C).

Heat the olive oil in a skillet over medium-high heat and sauté the onions and the celery seed until tender, about 5 minutes.

Add the garlic and sauté until fragrant, about a minute.

Add the diced tomatoes and parsley to the pan and sauté until most of the liquid is absorbed. Remove from heat and set aside.

Place the fish filets in a non-reactive baking pan or ceramic baker. Season them with salt and pepper and sprinkle with oregano on both sides. Top the fish fillets with the onion/celery/tomato mixture and cover each with two or three thin slices of lemon. In a small bowl, combine the lemon juice and the wine and pour over the fillets and into the pan. Top each of the fillets with panko. Bake the fillets uncovered for 30 to 40 minutes or until the fish flakes easily with a fork.

Sheet Pan Chicken Shawarma with Lemon Tahini Drizzle (GF)

Chicken

- 2 pounds boneless, skinless chicken thighs, chopped
- 1 TBL EVOO
- 2 garlic cloves minced
- ½ tsp Himalayan Sea salt
- ¾ tsp fresh ground black pepper
- ¼ tsp cayenne pepper
- 1 tsp ground cumin
- ½ tsp coriander
- ¼ tsp turmeric
- ¼ tsp ground cinnamon
- Grated zest of ½ organic lemon (1 tsp)
- 1 TBL fresh lemon juice

For the veggies: Approximately 8 cups total veggies-Any combo you like Suggestions:

- 1 ½ cups red onions, sliced (¾ medium)
- 2 medium red bell peppers, cut into ¼" slices (3 cups)
- Zucchini cut into slices (3 cups)
- Any other friendly veggies
- ¼ tsp Himalayan Sea salt
- ¼ tsp fresh ground black pepper
- 1 tsp dried oregano

Lemon-tahini drizzle

- 2 Tbsp Sunflower Tahini Sauce)
- 2 Tbsp EVOO
- 2 Tbsp fresh lemon juice (1 lemon)
- 2 TBL warm water
- 1 clove garlic minced
- ½ tsp honey

Preheat oven to 400°F (205°C) and line 2 large, rimmed baking sheets with parchment paper

Placed sliced chicken in large bowl and toss with evoo, garlic, salt, pepper, cayenne, cumin, coriander, turmeric, cinnamon, lemon zest, and lemon juice. Make sure everything is tossed evenly.

On one of the prepped baking sheets, place your veggies and add the evoo, salt, pepper and oregano.

On other prepared baking sheet, spread the chicken mixture in a single even layer. Transfer both sheet pans into the oven and bake for 20 to 25 until chicken is cooked through, and the veggies are just tender.

Meanwhile, in a small jar or container, combine all the drizzle ingredients and shake until well combined and set aside until ready to serve.

Serving Suggestions:

Chopped fresh herbs of choice to garnish

Lemon cut into wedges for serving

Steamed Fish with Ginger Snow Peas (GF)

- (1-inch) piece ginger, grated
- 2 cloves garlic, thinly sliced
- 6 scallions, sliced
- 4 (6-ounce) firm white fish fillets
- Sea salt and freshly ground pepper
- 4 tsp toasted sesame oil
- 1 Tbsp honey or agave
- ½ cup coconut aminos
- 2 Tbsp Chinese rice wine or dry sherry
- 1 pound snow peas, trimmed
- 4 cups spinach
- ½ cup shitakes chopped
- 2 Tbsp avocado oil

Set a large bamboo or metal steamer basket over a skillet of simmering water over medium heat.

Place the garlic and half each of the ginger and scallions on a plate that will fit inside the steamer. Score the fish skin a few times with a knife; season with salt and pepper. Place the fish skin-side up on the plate, mix honey with 2 teaspoons sesame oil and drizzle over fish. Put the plate in the steamer. Mix the coconut aminos and rice wine and pour over the fish.

Cover and steam the fish until just cooked through, 6 to 12 minutes, depending on the thickness. Carefully remove the hot plate.

In a medium pan over medium heat add the avocado oil and the rest of the ginger and snow peas. Sautee for one minute then add the shitakes and sauté for 3-4 minutes. Last add the spinach and sauté until it's lightly wilted, about one minute.

Transfer the vegetables to a platter, Top the vegetables with the fish and spoon the fish steamed juices on top and sprinkle with the remaining scallions.

Sweet & Spicy Steak Bites (GF)

- 1 small jalapeno
- 2 pounds of steak
- ½ tsp sea salt
- 2 Tbsp EVOO or Avocado Oil
- 2 Tbsp honey
- 1 tsp rice vinegar
- 1 medium line cut into eighths

Thinly slice 1 small jalapeno into rounds. Cut 1 lime into wedges. Cut the New York strip steak into 1-inch cubes and season with ½ teaspoon sea salt

Heat the 2 Tablespoons oil in a large skillet over medium-high heat until shimmering. Add steak cubes and sear until browned, flipping the halfway through. 6 to 8 minutes total. Add 2 Tablespoons honey, vinegar and the jalapeno and cook for 1 minute more. Remove from the heat and serve with the lime wedges.

Vegan Fried Rice (V) (GF)

- 3 Tbsp avocado oil
- 3 cups day old/cooled rice
- ¼ medium onion, diced
- 3 cloves garlic thinly sliced
- 1 cup kale, chopped
- 1 whole carrot diced
- 3 cups broccoli, chopped
- 3-4 shiitake mushrooms, chopped
- Salt & pepper
- 2 Tbsp gochujang (see page 133)
- 2 Tbsp coconut aminos
- 1 scallion, chopped
- 1 tsp sesame oil, optional
- 1 tsp sesame seeds, optional

Begin preparing the fried rice by mixing sauce—2 Tbsp gochujang and coconut aminos

Add 2 Tbsp v oil to a very large pan over highest heat setting. When oil begins to shimmer, add 1 cup of rice. Do not crowd the pan. Season with salt and pepper. Fry rice in oil until it starts to toast and remove and set aside. Repeat with remaining rice. Add 1 Tbsp of oil. Sautee all veggies in the sauce. Add rice and enjoy warm.

Vegan Thai Rice Stir Fry (V) (GF)

- 2 Tbsp evoo
- 2 Tbsp grated ginger
- 1 tsp chipotle
- 1 tsp cumin
- 1 tsp ground lemongrass
- 1 red onion, chopped
- 2 zucchini, chopped
- 2 yellow squash, chopped
- 4 carrots, chopped
- 2 cups snow peas, deveined
- 2 cup kale, deveined and chopped
- 1 cup haricots verts, chopped
- ½ cup water chestnuts
- 1 cup coconut milk
- 2 Tbsp honey
- 2 Tbsp sriracha
- 1 cup peanuts
- ½ cup mix of mint and basil leaves shredded
- Basmati rice for serving

Add evoo to a medium pan over low heat.

Add the spices and stir for one minute until fragrant. Add the vegetables and sauté for two minutes, then add the coconut milk, honey and sriracha. Sauté until vegetables are tender. Serve over rice and top with peanuts and basil/mix.

Vegetarian Meatballs

- 2 cups cooked wild rice
- 1 heaping cup finely chopped mushrooms
- ¼ cup chevre
- 2 eggs
- ¾ cup breadcrumbs
- 1 tsp onion powder
- 1 tsp garlic powder
- ½ tsp salt
- olive oil (optional)
- For the Gravy:
- 3 Tbsp salted butter
- ½ tsp onion powder and/or garlic powder
- 3 Tbsp flour
- 1 ½ cups vegetable broth
- ½ cup sour cream
- salt and black pepper to taste

Meatballs: Preheat the oven to 425°F (220°C). Mix the meatball ingredients together. Roll into 1-inch balls and place on a parchment-lined baking sheet. Bake for 15-20 minutes or until firm when you press them.

Gravy: Melt butter in a large skillet. Add onion powder, garlic powder, and flour. Let simmer until mixed thoroughly Slowly add broth, whisking after each addition, to make a smooth sauce. Stir in sour cream. Adjust consistency to taste with more broth. Season to taste.

Walnut Crusted Scallops (GF)

- ¼ to ⅓ cup unsalted walnuts
- ½ tsp garlic powder
- 12 to 16 oz Fresh Sea scallops
- ¼ tsp sea salt
- ¼ tsp fresh ground black pepper
- 2 Tbsp EVOO or avocado oil
- 1 Tbsp chopped parsley (TEST), or fresh basil for garnish or Green Onions or chives

Combine walnuts, garlic powder in large resealable food-storage bag and seal. Using meat mallet or back of skillet, crush the walnuts until they are a similar texture to panko breadcrumbs. Transfer to a large plate.

Spread the scallops in a single layer on paper towel and pat dry. Season both sides with salt and pepper.

In a large skillet, heat the oil over medium-high heat until it shimmers. Swirl the pan so the oil evenly coats the bottom. Dip both sides of each scallop into the walnut crumbs to coat each end like a crust. Working in batches so not to crowd the pan, add the scallops to the skillet. Cook until the scallops are golden brown on each side and cooked through, about 2 minutes per side. Transfer to paper -lined plate and repeat with remaining scallops

Sauces

Apricot Glaze (Spicy) (V) (GF)

- ½ cup Apricot Jam
- ¼ - ½ cup water
- Chipotle in Adobo Sauce- 1 Tbsp
- Option 2- smoked chipotle powder – 2 tsp (less sodium) available at Fairway

Combine all ingredients and blend until smooth. For a less spicy glaze, cut chipotle in adobo and chipotle powder to taste.

Blueberry Sauce (V) (GF)

- 2 shallots, peeled and very thinly sliced
- 1 ½ cups white wine
- 2 Tbsp Balsamic Vinegar
- 4 sprigs fresh thyme or rosemary
- 1 ⅓ cups blueberries (frozen can be used)
- OPTIONAL: 2 cinnamon sticks broken in half
- 4 Tbsp unsalted butter
- 2 Tbsp honey
- Black pepper to taste

In a medium saucepan over low heat, simmer together shallots, wine, vinegar, thyme, cinnamon if using and a pinch of sea salt until most of the liquid has evaporated, 15 to 20 minutes. Toss in the blueberries, butter and honey and cook until berries soften and turn the sauce pink-2 to 4 minutes

Chermoula (V) (GF)

- 3 Tbsp Evoo
- ½ cup basil
- ¼ cup mint
- ¼ cup oregano
- 4 garlic cloves, finely chopped
- 2 Tbsp lemon juice
- 2 tsp smoked chipotle powder
- 1 tsp ground cumin
- 1 tsp salt
- Pinch cayenne pepper, or more to taste (optional)
- Generous pinch saffron (optional)

Add all ingredients to a food processor and mix until smooth. Chermoula can be prepared up to 5 days in advance. Store in an airtight container in the fridge.

Gado Gado Sauce (V)

- • ¼ cup
- • 1 clove garlic (chopped)
- • 2 tbsp agave or honey
- • ½ tsp red curry paste
- • ¼ cup coconut milk
- • 2 tbsp fresh lime juice
- • 2½ tbsp coconut aminos
- • 2 tbsp water
- • 1 tsp fresh grated ginger
- • ¼ cup peanuts (crushed)

With the exception of the crushed peanuts, combine all the ingredients in a food processor and blend well. Remove the mixture from the processor and top the sauce with crushed peanuts.

Homemade Gochujang Paste (V) (GF)

- ½ cup white miso paste
- ⅓ cup Aleppo or Chipotle powder
- ¼ cup honey
- ¼ cup coconut aminos
- 1 tsp rice vinegar
- 1 tsp garlic powder
- 1 tsp onion powder

Place all ingredients in a mini food processor. Pulse until combined. Taste and adjust sweetness as needed. Store in an airtight container in the fridge for up to two weeks.

Indian Spice Rub (V) (GF)

- 6 Tbsp salt free curry powder
- ¼ tsp sea salt
- crushed red pepper or cayenne
- ground cumin
- ground coriander
- turmeric
- cinnamon
- ground ginger
- 1-2 Tbsp brown sugar

Combine ingredients. The ones that don't have a quantity- use a 6:1 ratio and adjust to taste. Store in airtight container- good for 4-6 months.

Lemon Goat Cheese Dipping Sauce (GF)

- 4 oz goat cheese
- 1 cup coconut milk
- 1 TBS chives
- ½ tsp black pepper
- ½ tsp lemon juice
- 1 tsp organic lemon zest

Place all ingredients except the lemon zest, in a food processor or blender and mix thoroughly.

Remove mixture from food processor and pour in bowl. Add lemon zest and mix.

Lyn-Genet Stir Fry Sauce (V) (GF)

- 4-inches fresh turmeric
- 4-inches fresh ginger
- 10 garlic cloves
- ¼ cup basil
- 1-3 chili peppers (optional) *You can sub cayenne, chipotle powder, cumin
- ¼ cup coconut aminos
- ¼ cup oil of choice (evoo, avocado, sesame)
- 2 Tbsp honey or agave

Blend everything up in a blender or food processor.

Peach Salsa (V) (GF)

- 2 cups of peaches diced
- ¼ cup minced red onion
- 2 tsp minced
- 2 Tbsp lime juice, more to taste
- Sea salt to taste

Place all of the ingredients in a bowl and stir to combine. Cover the bowl and refrigerate for at least 30 minutes or up to 1 day.

Plan Caesar (GF)

- 2 cloves garlic, chopped
- ¼cup evoo
- 4 oz goat cheese
- 2 Tbsp lemon juice
- 2tsp fresh black pepper
- 2 Tbsp fresh dill or basil, optional

Soak garlic cloves in evoo overnight. Add all ingredients to food processor with an S blade and blend until smooth. Add water as needed for lighter dressing.

Provençale Aioli Sauce (GF)

- 6 cloves of crushed garlic
- 2 egg yolks
- 1 cup Evoo
- 1 tsp lemon juice
- pinch of salt and pepper

In a bowl, whisk in the egg yolks and gradually add the olive oil until you make a mayonnaise-like sauce. Add in the crushed garlic, salt, pepper, and lemon juice, as you mix and whisk.

Quick Spicy Coco Sauce (V) (GF)

- 1 can coconut milk- do not use low fat please.
- 1 large onion
- 3-4 cloves of garlic
- spices: ginger, cinnamon, cumin, turmeric, black pepper and cayenne
- 1 Tbsp brown sugar

Sauté ginger, cinnamon, cumin, turmeric, garlic, onion, black pepper and cayenne- all to taste. Add ½ tsp salt and 1 heaping Tbsp brown sugar. Reduce for 20 min- will hold for 5 days or can freeze remainder. Portion is ⅛ cup per serving.

Simple Mango Chutney (V) (GF)

- 3 cups diced mango
- ½ cup finely diced red onion
- ⅓ cup brown sugar
- 5 Tbsp finely minced garlic
- 3 Tbsp finely minced ginger
- 3 Tbsp rice vinegar
- ¼ tsp salt
- ⅛ tsp cayenne

Combine all of the ingredients in a medium saucepan. Set over medium-low heat and cook, covered, for 30 minutes. Store in a sealed container.

Sunflower Tahini (V) (GF)

- 1 cup sunflower seeds
- ¼ cup extra virgin olive oil
- ¼ cup water
- 1 garlic clove, peeled
- 2 Tbsp lemon juice
- dash sea salt
- optional: add more water for creamier tahini

Add all ingredients to a food processor and blend until smooth, about 3 minutes.

Serve immediately, or store and refrigerate up to 5 days.

The Plan Hummus (V)

- 2 cups drained well-cooked or canned low sodium chickpeas; liquid reserved
- ¼ cup extra-virgin olive oil, plus oil for drizzling
- 2 cloves garlic, peeled
- Sea Salt and freshly ground black pepper to taste
- 1 Tbsp ground cumin, to taste, plus a sprinkling for garnish
- Juice of 1 lemon

Put everything except the parsley in a food processor and begin to process; add the chickpea liquid or water as needed to allow the machine to produce a smooth puree. Taste and adjust the seasoning (you may want to add more lemon juice).

Serve, drizzled with the olive oil and sprinkled with a bit more cumin

Thai Green Curry Paste (V) (GF)

- 1 tsp coriander
- 1 tsp cumin powder
- 1 tsp ground black pepper
- 3 small green chilies
- 5 cloves garlic, peeled
- 2 stalks lemongrass (tips trimmed, halved, + chopped)
- 1 heaping Tbsp fresh sliced ginger
- 6 stalks scallions
- 1 tsp ground turmeric
- ½ tsp sea salt (plus more to taste)
- 3 Tbsp lemon juice
- 3 Tbsp lime juice
- 1 Tbsp avocado oil
- 1 Tbsp honey
- 1 Tbsp coconut aminos

Add all ingredients to a food processor. The lemongrass will take a little time, just be patient. Taste and adjust flavors as needed. Refrigerate for up to one week.

Thai Red Curry Paste (V) (GF)

- 16 dried chilis
- 2 Tbsp lemongrass, sliced, reedy outer skin removed
- 1 Tbsp grated ginger or galangal
- 4 garlic cloves, peeled whole
- ½ tsp ground coriander
- ½ tsp ground cumin
- 1 Tbsp chopped Thai basil
- 2 garlic cloves
- 1 tsp organic lime zest
- ½ cup reserved chili soaking water

Place the chilies in a large bowl and pour over about 3 cups of freshly boiled water. Leave to soak for a good 30 minutes or so. Remove chilis and reserve water. Put chilis in a food processor. Add remaining curry paste ingredients and process well.

Vegan Alfredo Sauce (V) (GF)

- 1 cup raw cashew butter or raw cashew pieces
- ½ cup water
- ¼ cup evoo
- 2 garlic cloves, peeled
- ½ TBS lemon juice
- 1 tsp onion powder
- 2 TBS nutritional yeast
- ½ tsp sea salt
- ¼ tsp dried basil
- ¼ tsp black pepper

Blend everything together on high until creamy.

Sauce will stay in fridge up to 5 days or freeze.

Sauce will thicken as it's stored. If you want it thinner either add water or coconut milk for a super creamy sauce.

Zucchini Butter (V) GF

- 2 pounds zucchini or assorted summer squash (feel free to use less or add extra-cooking times will vary)
- ¼ cup EVOO
- 4 to 5 sprigs fresh thyme, rosemary or herb of choice OPTIONAL
- 2 minced shallots, garlic cloves, or combination of both
- ½ tsp sea salt
- ¼ tsp black pepper

Coarsely grate the zucchini and let it drain in a colander for 3 to 4 minutes or until you are ready to begin cooking. To hasten cooking time, squeeze the water out of the zucchini by wringing it in a clan cloth towel.

In a deep skillet, heat the olive oil/butter. Sauté the shallots or garlic briefly—don't let them brown. Add the zucchini and toss.

Cook and stir over medium to medium-high heat until the zucchini reaches a spreadable consistency, about 15 minutes.

Add the fresh herbs and salt and pepper after about 15 minutes. If the bottom of the pan is starting to scorch, turn the flame down! (Scrape those delicious bits into the butter for added flavor.) You can splash in a little water to help deglaze.

Desserts

Apple Pie Bread (GF)

- 2 cups blanched almond flour
- 1 Tbsp coconut flour
- 1 tsp ground cinnamon
- 1 tsp cardamom
- ½ tsp baking soda
- ¼ tsp cloves
- ¼ tsp sea salt
- ⅓ cup full fat coconut milk
- 4 Tbsp avocado oil
- 6 Tbsp honey

- 2 eggs
- ½ tsp vanilla extract
- 1 cup diced apples
- ⅓ cup pecans (chopped)

Crumb Topping:

- ¼ cup almond flour
- 1 tsp avocado oil
- ½ tsp cinnamon
- 1 Tbsp pecans (chopped)

Preheat oven to 350°F (175°C). Grease the bottom and sides of a 6.4 x 3.8-inch loaf pan with avocado oil, and line it with a piece of parchment paper. Cut paper to fit lengthwise, leaving some excess on the edges. You can also use an 8½ x 4½-inch medium loaf pan.

Mix the almond flour, coconut flour, cinnamon, cardamom, baking soda, cloves, and sea salt.

In a separate bowl, whisk together the coconut milk, avocado oil, honey, eggs, and vanilla extract.

Mix the dry and wet ingredients, just until combined. Do not over mix.

Gently fold the diced apple and chopped pecans into the batter. Pour the batter into the prepared loaf pan. In a bowl, mix all the crumb topping ingredients then sprinkle on batter.

Bake for approximately 45-50 minutes. Let bread cool. Remove the bread from the pan, slice, and serve warm.

Black and White Pound Cake (GF)

- 4 large eggs
- ½ cup avocado oil
- ½ cup sugar
- 1 tsp vanilla extract
- 1 Tbsp organic lemon zest or orange zest
- 2.5 cups blanched finely ground almond flour
- ¼ cup cocoa
- 1.5 tsp baking soda

Preheat your oven to 350°F (175°C). Oil a small loaf pan (8.5 X 4.5 inches). In a medium bowl, whisk the eggs, oil, sugar, baking soda and vanilla

Gradually add the lemon zest, almond flour. Mix cocoa to ⅓ the batter.

Alternate spooning in the cocoa batter and the plain batter in the pan. Bake the cake until golden and a toothpick inserted in its center comes out clean, roughly 30 minutes

Let cool and enjoy!

Cinnamon "Cream Cheese" Frosting (V)

- 1 cup raw cashew butter
- 3 Tbsp pure maple syrup
- 2 tsp lemon juice
- 2 tsp pure vanilla extract
- 1 tsp cinnamon
- 1 tsp cardamom
- ½ tsp nutmeg

Add the ingredients to a food processor and blend on high speed until smooth and creamy. Transfer the frosting to a bowl and chill in the refrigerator until it's ready to use.

Earl Grey Tea and Brandy Poached Pears (V) (GF)

- 2½ cups water
- 2 Earl Grey tea bags
- ⅓ cup agave
- 4 whole cloves
- 4 Tbsp brandy
- 4 medium firm-ripe pears
- Whipped cream, sorbet or ice cream (optional)

Bring the water to a boil in a large saucepan over high heat, then remove from the heat, add the tea bags, and let steep for 5 minutes. Discard the tea bags. Add the agave, cloves, and 3 Tbsp of the brandy: simmer.

Slice ½ inch off the bottom of each pear so that they will be able to stand upright.

Lay the pears on their sides in the tea, cover and cook for 7-10 minutes, turning the pears two or three times as they cook. Using a slotted spoon transfer the pears to a dish, standing upright.

Strain out the cloves. Increase the heat to medium-high and cook for about 10 minutes.

Remove from the heat; add the remaining Tbsp of brandy. Pour the sauce over the fruit.

Serve warm with optional toppings.

Lava Cakes

- 1 stick (4 ounces) unsalted butter
- 6 ounces bittersweet chocolate, preferably Valrhona
- 2 eggs
- 2 egg yolks
- ¼ cup sugar
- Pinch of salt
- 2 Tbsp all-purpose flour

Preheat the oven to 450°F (230°C). Butter and lightly flour four 6-ounce ramekins. Tap out the excess flour. Set the ramekins on a baking sheet.

In a double boiler, over simmering water, melt the butter with the chocolate. In a medium bowl, beat the eggs with the egg yolks, sugar and salt at high speed until thickened and pale.

Whisk the chocolate until smooth. Quickly fold it into the egg mixture along with the flour. Spoon the batter into the prepared ramekins and bake for 12 minutes, or until the sides of the cakes are firm but the centers are soft. Let the cakes cool in the ramekins for 1 minute, then cover each with an inverted dessert plate. Carefully turn each one over, let stand for 10 seconds and then unmold. Serve immediately.

Lavender Simple Syrup

- 1 cup water
- 2 Tbsp dried lavender
- ½ cup agave or honey

Add all the ingredients to a small saucepan and bring to a boil. Turn down the heat and simmer for 20 minutes.

Remove the pan from the heat and strain the flowers.

Let cool and transfer to glass container.

Keep refrigerated.

Lemon Ice Cream (V) (GF)

- 1 can coconut milk
- 3 lemons (remove zest and rind if you wish)
- ¼ cup maple syrup

Put the mixture in a high-speed blender and give it a quick whirl and then pour into ice cube tray. Let the lemon mixture freeze. Take mixture out of freezer and let gently thaw for a few minutes before throwing back in the blender. Give the blender a good hard blend until it becomes creamy. You can then enjoy the fruits of your labor or freeze in a tub.

Raspberry Truffles (V) (GF)

- ¼ cup coconut milk
- 7 oz vegan chocolate chips
- 23 ml (½ Tbsp) framboise (raspberry brandy), optional
- 170 grams (6 ounces) fresh raspberries
- 120 ml (½ cup) unsweetened cocoa powder

Line a rimmed baking sheet with waxed paper and set aside.

In a small heavy saucepan, over medium heat, bring the milk just to a simmer. Remove from the heat and stir in the chopped chocolate until smooth. Add the framboise, if using, and stir to combine.

Pat berries dry. Add a handful of berries to the chocolate in the saucepan and use a rubber spatula to gently coat them with the chocolate. Remove berries, one at a time and let cool. Place on a baking sheet or plate.

Place the sheet into the refrigerator and chill for at least 1 hour, until the chocolate is firm.

Drizzle berries with cocoa powder.

Swedish Cardamom-Blackberry Linzer Cookies

- 2 cups all-purpose flour
- 1 cup raw almonds
- 2 to 3 tsp ground cardamom
- ¼ tsp salt
- 1 cup unsalted butter, softened
- ½ cup plus 1 tsp sugar, divided
- 1 large egg
- 1 cup chia jam (page 73)
- 1 Tbsp lemon juice
- 3 Tbsp confectioners' sugar

In a food processor, combine ½ cup flour and almonds; pulse until almonds are finely ground. Add cardamom, salt and remaining flour, Pulse until combined.

In a large bowl, cream butter and ½ cup sugar until light and fluffy. Beat in egg. Gradually beat in flour mixture.

Divide dough in half. Shape each into a disk; wrap in plastic. Refrigerate 1 hour or until firm enough to roll.

Preheat oven to 350°F (175°C).

On a lightly floured surface, roll each portion to ⅛-in. thickness. Cut with a floured 2-in. round cookie cutter. Using a floured 1-in. round cookie cutter, cut out the centers of half of the cookies. Place solid and window cookies 1 in. apart on greased baking sheets. Bake 10-12 minutes or until light brown.

Remove from pans to wire racks to cool completely. In a small bowl, mix chia jam, lemon juice and remaining sugar. Spread filling on bottoms of solid cookies, Top with window cookies. Dust with confectioners' sugar.

Made in United States
North Haven, CT
25 February 2022